THE TARDIEU SERIES

the essentials in
cardiac pacing

GUY FONTAINE, M.D.

Laboratory of Clinical Electrophysiology
La Salpêtrière and Fernand-Widal Hospitals
Paris

YVES GROSGOGEAT, M.D.

Professor of Cardiology
La Salpêtrière Hospital
Paris

JEAN-JACQUES WELTI, M.D.

Professor of Cardiology
Fernand-Widal Hospital
Paris

BERNARD TARDIEU

Medical Illustrator

Foreword by Victor Parsonnet, M.D.

Director of Surgery
Newark Beth Israel Medical Center
New Jersey Medical School
Newark, N.J.

1978
MARTINUS NIJHOFF MEDICAL DIVISION — THE HAGUE
LONDON — BOSTON

MARTINUS NIJHOFF MEDICAL DIVISION, 160 Old Derby Street, Hingham, MA 02043, U.S.

ISBN-13: 978-90-247-2102-3   e-ISBN-13: 978-94-009-9736-3
DOI: 10.1007/978-94-009-9736-3

FOREWORD

The classic medical textbook tends to be overly technical, excessively detailed, profusely referenced, and the antithesis of enjoyable reading. With the expectation of many hours of hard work, I was unprepared for the pleasure that lay ahead.

This book is what we in the United States call a « sleeper ». Without pomp or solemnity it captures you with a light-hearted style that subtly belies its sophistication. The authors have indeed mastered the art of simplicity, combining profound knowledge with an airy format, to a degree that is hard to emulate. All the salient features of pacing are presented here, from history and pathology to complications and long-range follow-up. Perhaps it is a mark of excellence, rather than a confession of my personal ignorance, to say that there is scarcely a section that did not provide me with a new bit of information or a new insight.

Permanent pacing of the heart is so common nowadays, at least in the more affluent sections of the world, that almost every person must know of someone with an implanted pacemaker. In the United States, where there are more than 100,000 new implants each year, almost every sizeable hospital has a pacemaker implantation service and almost every physician in a related field is interested in doing this surgery. All that should really be required is that the surgeon make himself an expert. This book, if thoroughly understood, will provide the expertise, and reading it will be a labor of love. The illustrations are laced with humor and charm, and the text will appeal to almost any reader.

After reviewing the first edition I had urged the authors to prepare an American version because I believed the book to be extremely valuable not only to the beginner in pacing, but to the more experienced physician as well. This second edition has added new illustrations and information on the most recent technical advances, and there is also an expanded reference list. The authors present solid reasoning for all of their concepts and methods of practice, and give food for thought even to those whose opinions may differ slightly. It is my hope to see still later editions of this delightful book in years to come.

Victor Parsonnet, M.D.
Director of Surgery
Newark Beth Israel Medical Center
New Jersey Medical School
Newark, N.J.

TABLE OF CONTENTS

IMPLANTATION OF PACEMAKERS

PREFACE

A pacemaker is an implanted electronic device which takes over command of the cardiac rhythm when the natural mechanism fails. In practical terms, it consists of a battery, and an electronic circuit which transforms the continuous electric current into short electrical impulses. The rhythm of the myocardium will be that imposed by these impulses which are therefore regulated at 70-80/min (lasting about 1/1000 second each with an amplitude in the order of several volts). The whole device is enclosed in a sealed case made out of metal or epoxy-resin. The electrical impulses are conducted to the heart muscle by isolated electrodes and depolarisation of the heart follows the minute electrical discharge which takes place at the tip of the electrodes. **Depolarisation** leads to contraction of the ventricular muscle.

The main use of the pacemaker has been in the treatment of Stokes-Adams' syndrome, a permanent slow pulse or atrio-ventricular block, the prognosis of which has been completely changed. Formerly, half the patients with this disease died within a year of diagnosis. Now-adays, with a pacemaker, the expectation of life of these patients is practically the same as for people of the same age without the disease.

Pacemakers have been used in the treatment of other cardiac irre-gularities giving rise to syncope and even for symptomatic simple brady-cardias. Recent uses include the treatment of tachycardia-bradycardia syndromes and prevention of certain tachycardias.

A pacemaker was first implanted in man in 1958. V. Parsonnet during the Vth International Symposium in Tokyo (1976) stated that there are now about 156,000 patients with permanent pacemakers in the United States alone and we estimate the world population of pacemaker patients to be about 300,000. The therapeutic results achieved by these devices are among the most spectacular of modern medicine. Pacemakers are in certain cases, the only means of maintaining human life from second to second throughout many years.

7

PHYSIOLOGY OF
THE INTRACARDIAC CONDUCTION SYSTEM

The structure and function of cardiac muscle is unique. It is striated muscle, not directly under control of the central nervous system and quite independant of voluntary control. It does not tetanise. It has an inherent automatism and contracts in a constant predetermined manner.

These singular properties are better understood by study of the individual myocardial cells. Recent advances have increased our knowledge of the physiology and pathology of the intracardiac conduction system, the essentials of which are outlined below.

A) CELLULAR ELECTROPHYSIOLOGY

1. Resting potential

Each myocardial cell is enclosed in a lipo-protein cytoplasmic membrane (Plate II, p 12). The ionic concentrations are different on each side of this membrane. In the resting state, there is a higher concentration of potassium ions inside the cell than in the interstitial fluid. Sodium ions are more abundant in the interstitial fluid. The **ionic gradients** across the cell membrane are responsible for the resting electrical potential of the cell, the exterior being positively charged with respect to the interior. If a micro-electrode is introduced into the resting myocardial cell, a potential of — 90 millivolts will be recorded with reference to the interstitial fluid.

The myocardial cell is **excitable,** that is to say that if a mechanical, chemical or electrical stimulus is applied at a site on the cell membrane, the polarisation will be disturbed and this change of polarisation will be propagated all along the cell membrane. The external charge becomes negative and the internal positive. This change in potential may be recorded with a micro-electrode producing a characteristic trace known as the **action potential.**

2. Action potential

Activation of the resting myocardial cell suddenly changes the internal potential from — 90 millivolts to + 20 millivolts. This is the phase of rapid depolarisation (Phase 0). At the same time, ionic transfers occur with a sudden influx of sodium ions into the cell and an efflux of potassium ions from inside the cell. This is followed by a plateau phase (Phases 1 and 2), attributed to a slow flow of sodium and calcium ions into the cell. A recovery phase with a return to the resting potential of — 90 millivolts which remains stable until the next depolarisation then occurs (Phase 4). Repolarisation to the resting

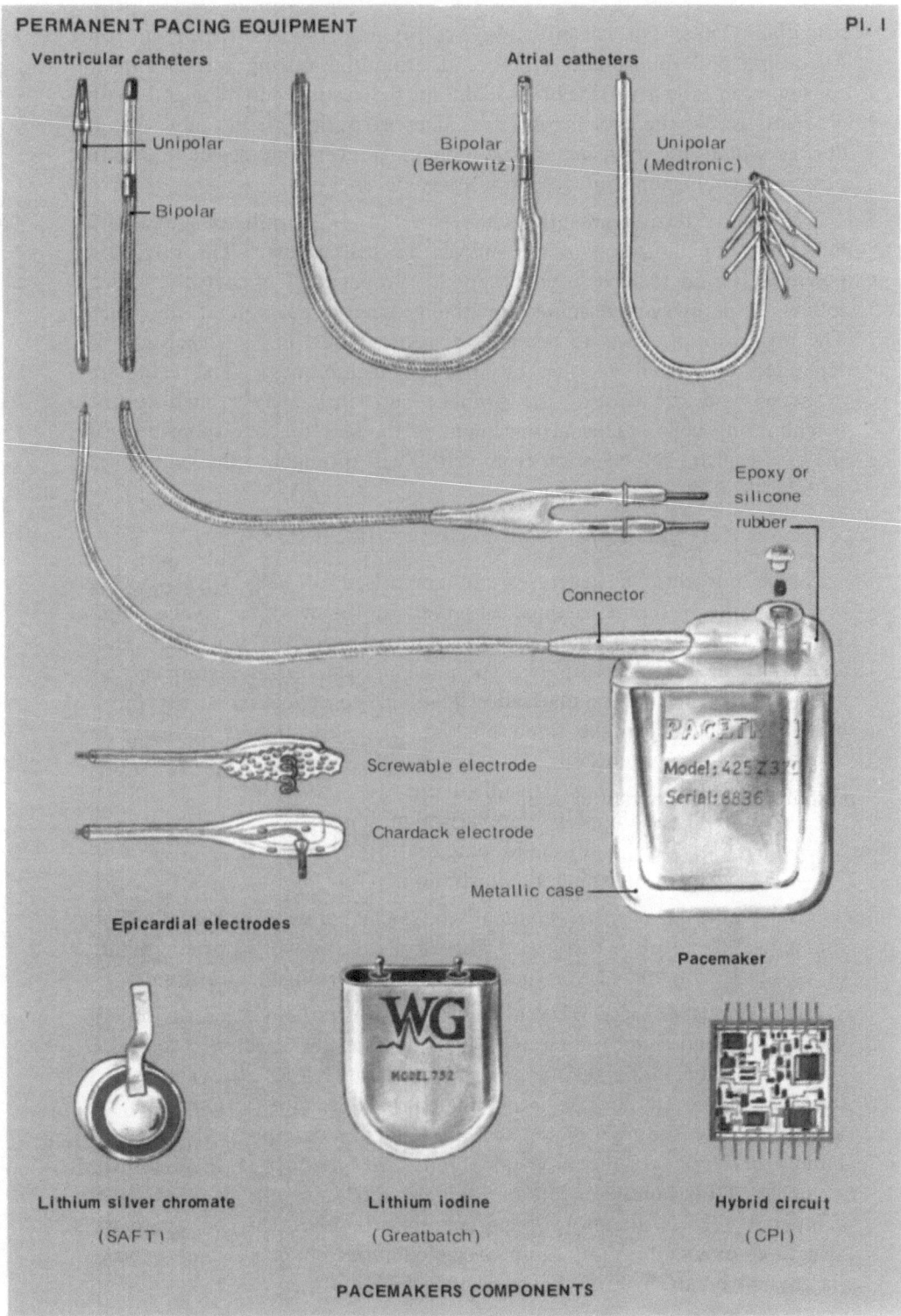

Ventricular catheters

Unipolar

Bipolar

Atrial catheters

Bipolar (Berkowitz)

Unipolar (Medtronic)

Epoxy or silicone rubber

Connector

Screwable electrode

Chardack electrode

Epicardial electrodes

Metallic case

PACETR...
Model: 425 Z37...
Serial: 8836

Pacemaker

Lithium silver chromate
(SAFT)

WG
MODEL 732
Lithium iodine
(Greatbatch)

Hybrid circuit
(CPI)

PACEMAKERS COMPONENTS

Tardieu

potential (Phase 3) is an energy consuming process dependant on Adenosine 5'-Triphosphate (ATP). During the resting phase, energy consumption is just sufficient to maintain the resting potential and ionic gradients across the cell membranes. Depolarisation on the other hand, during which the transmembrane potentials even out seems to be a passive phenomenon and does not consume energy.

When the resting potential changes from — 90 millivolts to — 60 millivolts, depolarisation of the myocardial cell occurs. The **threshold potential** is said to have been attained. Propagation of activation then follows a pathway determined by the geometric position of the cells. The myocardium seems to act as a syncytium but, in fact, each cell is separated one from another by the cell membranes. The cells are Y-shaped and the tips of the branches are intimately related to the neighbouring cells. This arrangement is thought to be responsible for the easy transfer of activation from cell to cell throughout the ventricular muscle.

3. **Action potential of pacemaker cells**

Some intracardiac structures are comprised of cells whose action potentials are different to those observed in the working myocardium. Their rate of depolarisation is slower, there is no plateau phase and, above all, the time between two spontaneous depolarisations appears as a long phase of **slow depolarisation** leading spontaneously to the threshold potential. Then the rapid phase of depolarisation is observed as in the working myocardium. In this type of cell, "automatism" is said to exist. This property is dependant on:
   —The slope of the slow depolarisation phase;
   —The level of the threshold potential;
   —The level of maximal repolarisation.

The whole intracardiac conduction system varies only slightly from this pattern from place to place. These cells also have a slowed rhythm of depolarisation the nearer they are to the working myocardium.

The sino-atrial node (Keith and Flack) has the fastest rhythm at 70/min and under normal circumstances acts as the cardiac pacemaker. If the S-A node fails then the atrio-ventricular node (Tawara) takes over command (these cells are situated between the atrium and the atrial roots of the A-V node and the junction of the node and the bundle of His). If the A-V node fails, the conductive tissue of the branches of the bundle of His or even the Purkinje cells may take over command. It is therefore apparant that a **hierarchy** of automatic structures exists, the most rapid of which takes command and imposes its rhythm on the rest of the heart muscle.

4. Excitability of the myocardial cell

If the excitability of a myocardial cell is studied using an electrical stimulus just strong enough to depolarise the cell (threshold stimulus) the amplitude of the stimulus needed to obtain activation remains constant during the interval between two depolarisations of the same cell. This is called the **diastolic threshold.** If the stimulus is applied earlier in the cycle, near the end of the action potential, a depolarisation may be obtained with a weaker stimulus. This is known as the **supernormal phase.** It is situated near the end of the T-wave of the surface ECG. If the stimulus is advanced even earlier, that is to say during the repolarisation phase, it is still possible to obtain depolarisation but with a stronger stimulus. This is the **relative refractory period** which corresponds to the summit of the T-wave. If a strong stimulus is applied during this period, the myocardial cells, at different stages of repolarisation may be activated in an asynchronous fashion leading to ventricular fibrillation.

Stimulation earlier still in the cycle is unable to elicit a response as it falls in the **absolute refractory period.**

B) INTRACARDIAC CONDUCTION

The cardiac rhythm is normally determined by the **sino-atrial node,** that is to say the conductive tissue with the fastest automatic activity. The node is situated in the upper part of the right atrium near the point of entry of the superior vena cava (Plate III, p 16).

After depolarising the atrium, the activation arrives at the **node of Tawara** or atrio-ventricular (A-V) node on the opposite side of the atrium. This is the first part of the atrio-ventricular conduction system. Its structure is unique, the histology resembling an intermediate between cardiac muscle and nervous tissue. It is separated from the neighbouring myocardium by a band of collagen tissue. The A-V node is situated on the right side of the inter-ventricular septum more or less parallel to the site of insertion of the septal leaflet of the tricuspid valve. The time delay for the activation to arrive at the A-V node from the S-A node is in the order of 70 ms. At this point, the activation is suddenly slowed, taking about 60 ms to cross the 1 cm length of the A-V node. It is then conducted to the **bundle of His** which crosses the septal leaflet of the tricuspid valve and follows the crest of the inter-ventricular septum for 1·5 to 2 cm.

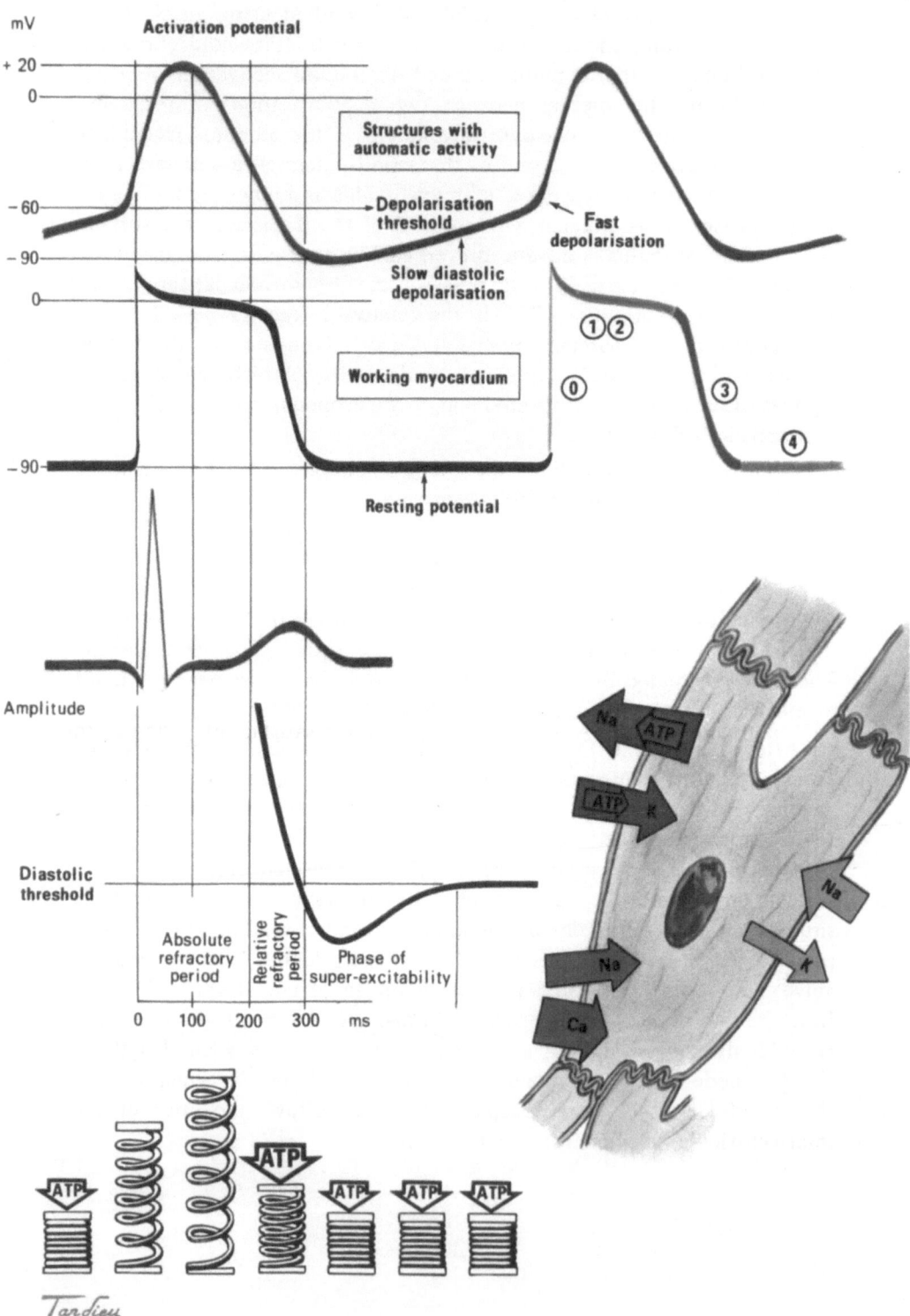

mV **Activation potential**

+ 20

0

Structures with
automatic activity

− 60 Depolarisation
threshold

− 90 Slow diastolic
depolarisation

0

Working myocardium

Fast
depolarisation

① ②

⓪

③

④

− 90 Resting potential

Amplitude

Diastolic
threshold

Absolute
refractory
period

Relative
refractory
period

Phase of
super-excitability

0 100 200 300 ms

Na ATP

ATP K

Na

Na

K

Ca

ATP

ATP

ATP ATP ATP

Tardieu

12

The bundle of His divides into a long narrow right branch which activates the endocardium of the right ventricle. On the left side, the bifurcation gives rise to a wide thick left bundle which itself branches to activate the endocardium of the left ventricle. These branches are schematically represented as the **antero-superior** and **postero-inferior** fascicles. They terminate in the same manner as the right bundle, in the numerous branches of the **Purkinje system** which therefore forms the intermediate between the branches of the bundle of His and the ventricular muscle. The conduction interval between the trunk of the bundle of His and the start of ventricular activation is about 40 ms.

This pathway (A-V node, bundle of His and branches) is the only way that atrial depolarisation may normally be conducted to the ventricles as the atrial and ventricular muscles form two isolated electrical entities. Slowing of conduction at the A-V node allows time for satisfactory filling of the ventricles before their contraction. Conduction in the branches of the bundle of His is 4-5 times more rapid than in myocardial muscle so ensuring an activation sequence of the ventricles from the endocardium outwards, giving the optimal haemodynamic result.

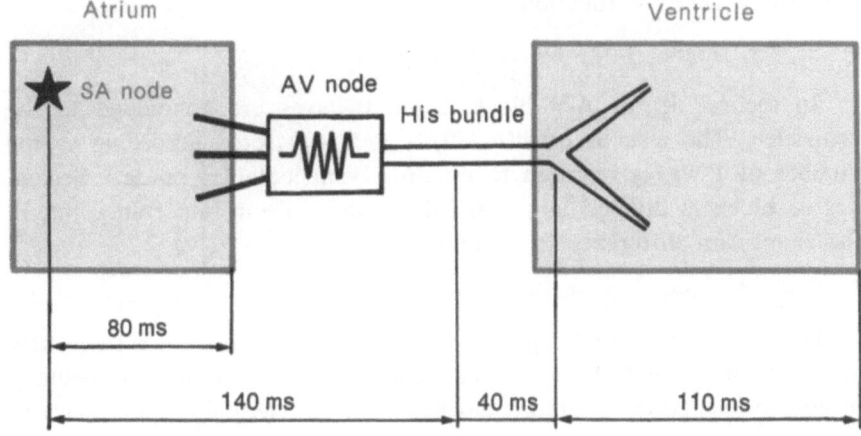

INTRACARDIAC CONDUCTION DEFECTS

A) ATRIO-VENTRICULAR CONDUCTION DEFECT

By nature of the activation of the heart from the sinus node to the contractile ventricle, any disease process involving the A-V node, bundle of His or its branches, if sufficiently diffuse, may interrupt the conduction to the ventricle. This is the situation in **atrio-ventricular block,** a more precise term for the **Stokes-Adams syndrome.**

1. Third degree atrio-ventricular block

Third degree A-V block is said to be present when there is **no transmission** of atrial activity to the ventricle (Plate V, p 21). In the absence of the pacing rhythm of the sinus node, command is taken over by more distal cells of the conduction system of a slower automatism. The slower rhythm arises distal to the zone blocked, either in the branches of the bundle of His or in the Purkinje system. In the latter case, which is the most frequently encountered, the ventricles beat at about 40/min. This is called **idio-ventricular** rhythm and is asynchronous with the beating of the atria which continue at the rhythm of the S-A node. The rate of the idio-ventricular rhythm is half that of sinus rhythm and it is not affected by effort. Its remarkable stability led to the term **permanent slow pulse** previously applied to the Stokes-Adams syndrome. Idio-ventricular rhythm may be considered as a safety device but is itself susceptible to failure. In this case, another more distal group of cells may take over command at an equal or even slower rate and with a different ECG morphology (the point of origin in the ventricle is different). If these secondary pacemakers all fail, syncopal episodes will occur. Even at a rate of 40/min, the cardiac output is reduced, causing symptoms such as shortness of breath on exertion and tiredness, and in the older persons, heart failure and diminished cerebral function.

2. Second degree atrio-ventricular block

In second degree A-V block, **some P-waves** are conducted to the ventricle. The term is qualified 2/1, 3/1, 4/1, etc., according to the number of P-waves required to obtain a ventricular response. Second degree block is divided into two sub-groups. Their importance lies in the significant difference in prognosis.

a) Type I (Wenckebach)

In this type of second degree A-V block, the P-R interval is frequently longer than normal. It is **not constant** from beat to beat showing a progressive lengthening until a blocked P-wave. The delay takes place in most cases in the A-V node and it is thought that the P-wave which does not elicit a ventricular response is also blocked at this level. This is not the most dangerous type of block as the bundle of His may take over the pacing role should the process aggravate, so avoiding cardiac arrest.

b) **Type II** (Mobitz)

This type of second degree A-V block is characterised by the fact that the P-wave conducted is **constant** and followed by QRS complex after a frequently normal P-R interval. This type of block is usually situated in the bundle of His. It is associated with a poorer prognosis than nodal blocks as it may lead abruptly to complete heart block and sudden death may occur.

c) **Luciani-Wenckebach period**

This is a special type I second degree A-V block characterised by **periodic** lengthening of the P-R interval through several cardiac cycles until a P-wave is not followed by a ventricular response. This type of conduction defect is also generally due to a block in the A-V node.

3. **First degree heart block**

This is the least severe form of atrio-ventricular conduction defect in which there is a delay of conduction from the atrium to the ventricle. Each P-wave is followed by a ventricular response, the ECG showing a long fixed P-R interval.

4. **Clinical consequences**

Atrio-ventricular blocks may be paroxistic, the **ECG being completely normal** between attacks. Great care is therefore required when faced with a patient of over 60 years of age presenting with syncopal episodes. Stokes-Adams attacks must be considered in the differential diagnosis before attributing the symptom to a neurological or functional illness. One must also be vigilant when dealing with patients presenting with symptoms varying from lightheadedness, vertigo, tinnitus and unsteadiness to "sudden turns" without loss of consciousness. In some cases, complete heart block does not present with syncope but with shortness of breath on exertion and tiredness.

Diagnosis is easily made when the pulse rate is slow and the ECG shows a high grade A-V block. However, it may be more difficult in the early stages of the illness when the ventricle is dependant or partially so on sinus rhythm. A practically normal A-V conduction may be present.

Usually, however, progression to complete block is preceeded by diffuse disease of the intra-ventricular system which gives rise to particular ECG abnormalities. It is important to be able to recognize these in order to make the correct diagnosis and consider the indications for the implantation of a pacemaker.

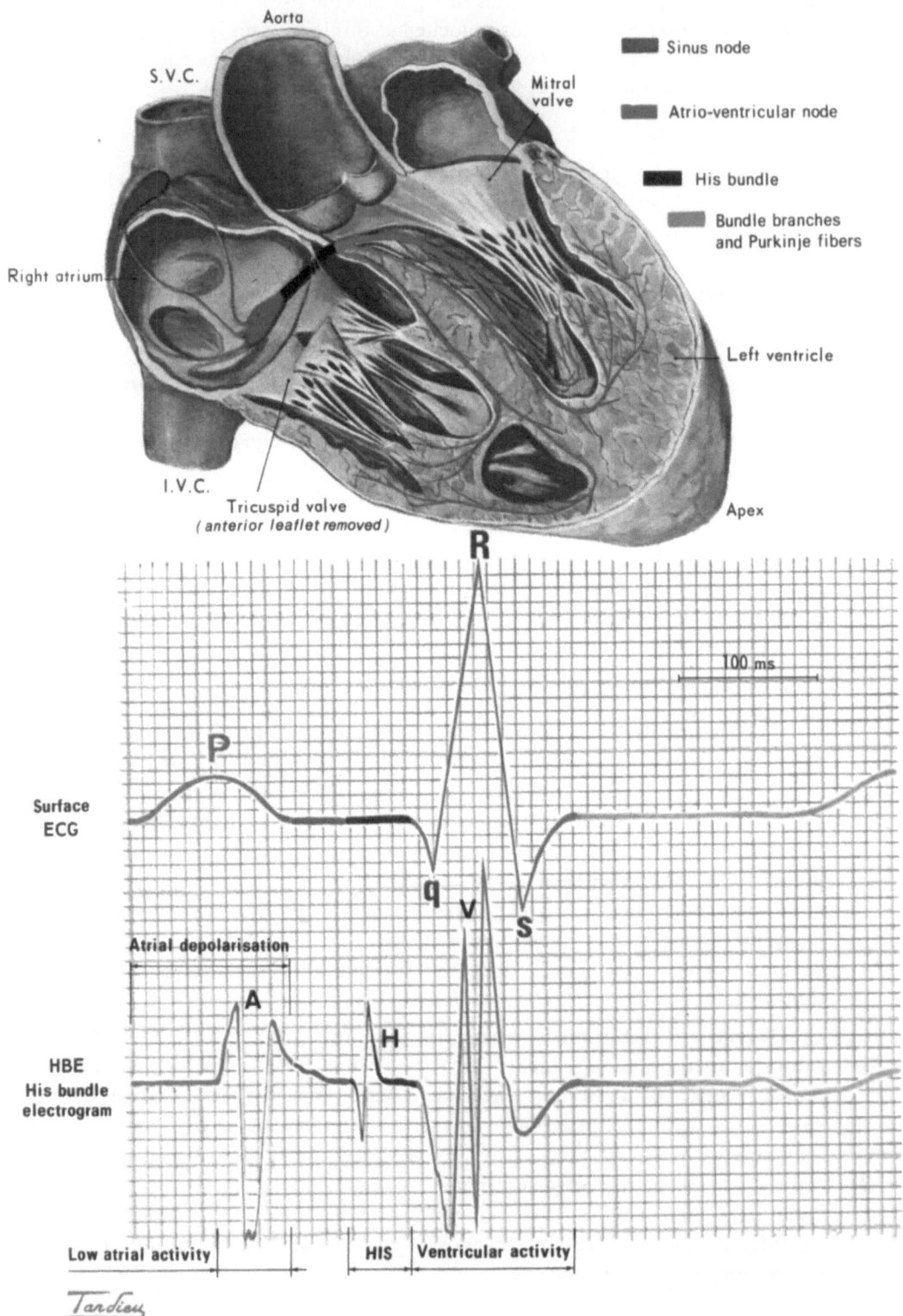

Aorta

S.V.C.

Mitral valve

Sinus node

Atrio-ventricular node

His bundle

Bundle branches and Purkinje fibers

Right atrium

Left ventricle

I.V.C.

Tricuspid valve
(anterior leaflet removed)

Apex

R

100 ms

P

Surface
ECG

q
V
s

Atrial depolarisation

A

H

HBE
His bundle
electrogram

Low atrial activity   HIS   Ventricular activity

Tardieu

16

B) INTRA-VENTRICULAR CONDUCTION DEFECTS

1. Bundle branch blocks

The details of right and left bundle branch blocks, recordings of which are shown in the suitable figure (Plate IV, p 20), are omitted so that segmental conduction defects may be explained at greater length.

2. Fascicular or segmental blocks

Conduction defects arising from the antero-superior or postero-inferior fascicles, may be recognized from the surface ECG (see figures). Left fascicular conduction defects may be associated with right bundle conduction defects, the so-called **bi-blocks**. The anatomy of the fascicles has a prognostic significance. The antero-superior fascicle is narrower and more easily damaged than the wide postero-inferior fascicle. Right bundle branch blocks associated with posterior hemi-block progress more frequently to complete heart block than a right bundle branch block with a left anterior hemi-block. Conduction may alternate between the fascicles and two hemi-blocks may be recorded in the same patient on the same tracing.

In different recordings a right bundle branch block may be associated with firstly a left anterior hemi-block and then with a left posterior hemi-block, so called **trifascicular block.**

Finally, these intra-ventricular conduction defects may be **associated** with varying degrees of A-V conduction defects, so allowing the determination of the site and nature of the block from the surface ECG. These cases are relatively rare. Patients with A-V or intra-ventricular conduction defects may suddenly and without any warning develop complete heart block giving rise to the most serious complication of this disease, syncope.

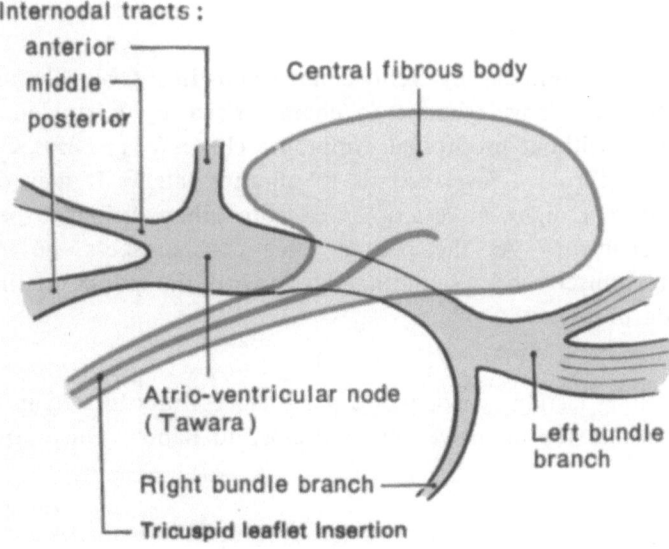

17

SYNCOPES

A) CLINICAL FEATURES

1. Ventricular standstill

Complete heart block may occur without ventricular escape rhythm and result in ventricular standstill with circulatory arrest. If this situation lasts more than a few seconds, symptoms of acute cerebral anoxia will result with loss of consciousness or syncope. The cardiac arrest may last seconds or minutes before ending in most cases in a ventricular escape rhythm. As the circulation is reestablished, the patient regains colour and full consciousness (Plate VI, p 25).

2. Tachycardias-Fibrillation

Under certain conditions, a rate of 40/min predisposes to uneven repolarisation and a burst of two or three ventricular extrasystoles may trigger a tachycardia called "**Torsade de pointes**" (Plate VIII, p 29) or even ventricular fibrillation. In these situations, ventricular activation is fast and poorly synchronised, leading to a fall in cardiac output and syncope. In most cases, the tachycardia stops spontaneously after a few seconds and an idio-ventricular rhythm or even normal A-V conduction is reestablished.

If however ventricular standstill or tachycardia last more than a few minutes, anoxia may lead to irreversible cerebral damage and death. There is no way of knowing in a patient with A-V block if the first syncope will be fatal. This is the rationale for the implantation of a pacemaker as a routine in these patients. Many patients however remain well throughout many years with paroxystic or more especially idiopathic heart blocks, but at the present time, there is no way of differentiating these from the others.

3. Stokes-Adams syncopes

Whether precipitated by ventricular standstill or by "Torsades de pointes" Stokes-Adams syncope is characterised by a sudden loss of consciousness without prodromal symptoms (Plate VI, p 25). Complete recovery is the rule a few seconds to minutes later. It may occur at any time, day or night, at rest or on exertion, there being no particular trigger mechanism. As the patient loses consciousness, he may fall so injuring himself and simulating death with the pupil dilating after 10 seconds of so.

—*Cardiac massage* (Plate VII, p 27)

Severe long lasting syncopes are most successfully treated in hospital where resources for intensive care are close to hand. Once circulatory arrest has been diagnosed by the **absence of the femoral pulse,** external cardiac massage should be started. The sternum is depressed (with both hands, one on top of the other) at a rhythm of 40-50/min. The amount of pressure applied is critical; if it is too light, the massage will be ineffective; if it is too heavy, there will be a risk of fracturing ribs or costochondral joints. The efficiency of the massage may be determined by palpation of the femoral pulse. External cardiac massage is sometimes sufficient to restart ventricular standstill. The patient will flush as he regains consciousness. In other cases, massage may be followed by other resuscitatory measures.

—External electrical countershock (Plate VIII, p 29)

An ECG tracing is essential during cardiac arrest to know whether the patient is in **ventricular fibrillation** or **asystole.** There are no clinical signs to distinguish the two. Asystole is treated by external cardiac massage and an infusion of **isoprenaline.** When "Torsades de pointes" are present, it is a mistake to countershock too soon as it is known that many stop spontaneously. Certain authors think that electric shocks upset ionic gradients at cellular level so predisposing to further arrhythmias.

If the patient has lost consciousness, an electrical countershock is applied. It is often necessary to continue external cardiac massage after the arrhythmia has been stopped as it is often replaced by a slow unstable idio-ventricular rhythm. This slow rhythm may be interrupted by bigeminal and trigeminal ventricular extrasystoles which may trigger another ventricular tachycardia. In this case, an intravenous infusion of **isoprenaline** is indicated to speed up the idio-ventricular rhythm and so abolish the syncopal state.

If ventricular standstills recur and isoprenaline is ineffective or the tachycardias poorly controlled, **temporary pacing** is indicated without delay.

B) TECHNIQUES FOR TEMPORARY PACING

The two main complications of temporary pacing are infection and displacement of the tip of the pacing catheter. The risk of these complications may be minimised by operating in a catheter room or a sterile operating theatre equiped for radiological screening and by the possession of **good operative technique.**

1. Femoral approach (Plate IX, p 33)

The patient is shaved and the skin disinfected with iodine. The patient is completely covered with sterile towels, especially the legs on which the pacing catheter will be placed during manipulation of the

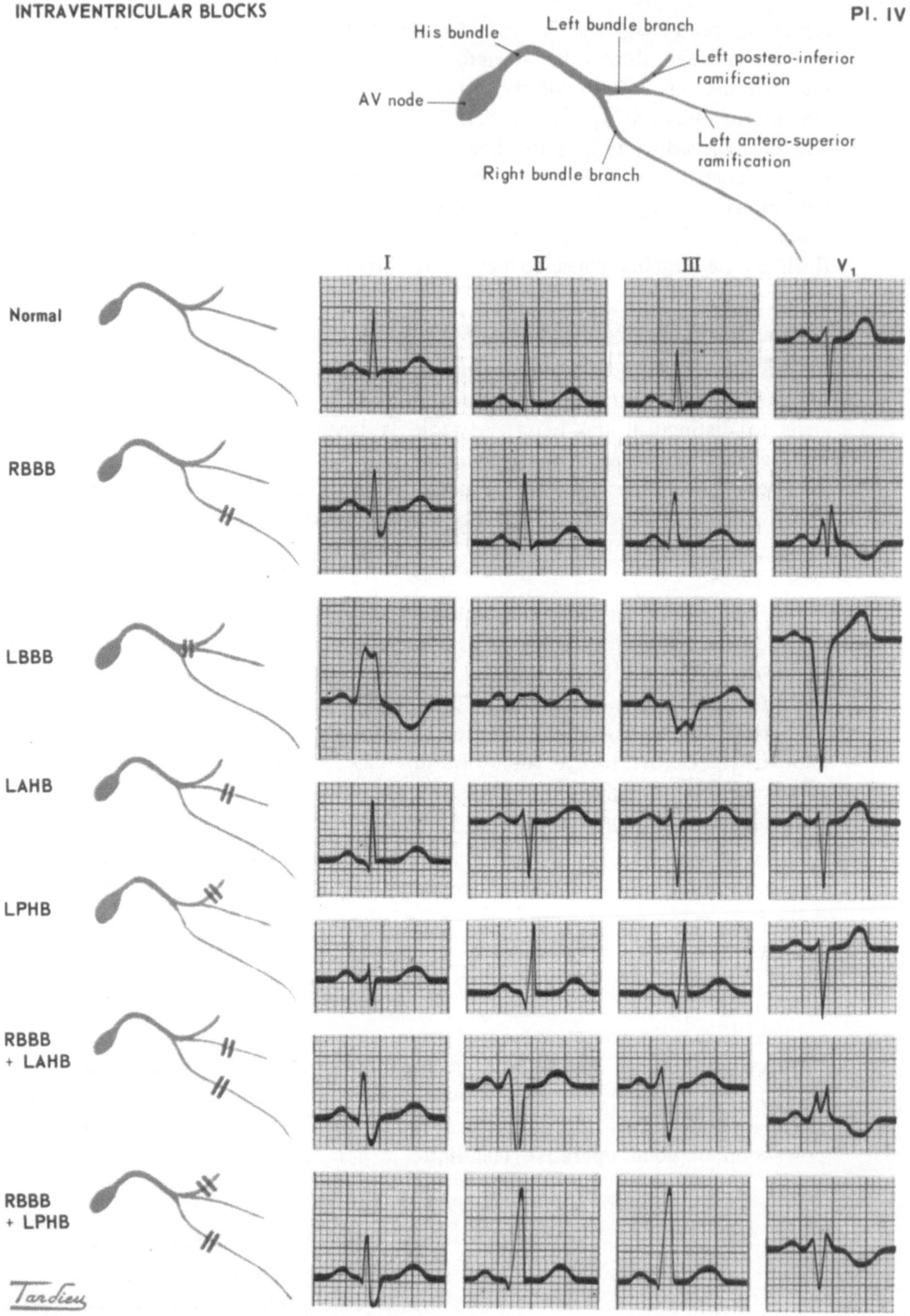

Pl. IV

His bundle

Left bundle branch

Left postero-inferior ramification

AV node

Left antero-superior ramification

Right bundle branch

I II III V₁

Normal

RBBB

LBBB

LAHB

LPHB

RBBB + LAHB

RBBB + LPHB

Tardieu

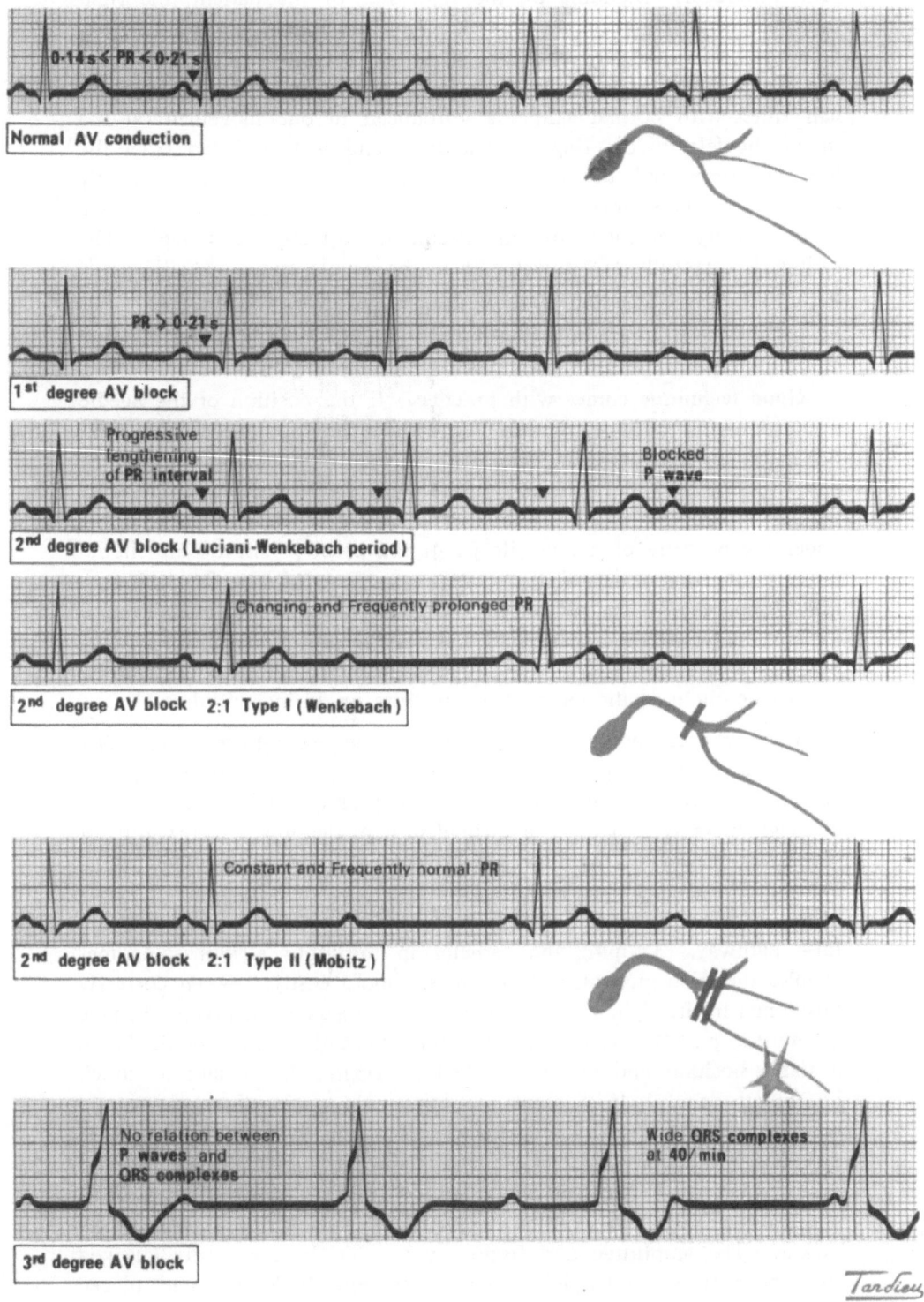

Normal AV conduction

0·14 s < PR < 0·21 s

1st degree AV block

PR > 0·21 s

2nd degree AV block (Luciani-Wenkebach period)

Progressive lengthening of PR interval

Blocked P wave

2nd degree AV block 2:1 Type I (Wenkebach)

Changing and Frequently prolonged PR

2nd degree AV block 2:1 Type II (Mobitz)

Constant and Frequently normal PR

3rd degree AV block

No relation between P waves and QRS complexes

Wide QRS complexes at 40/min

Tardieu

vein introducer. Standing on the right side of the patient, the right inguinal ligament is located. The skin puncture is performed 3-4 finger-breadths below. Firstly, the femoral artery is controlled by the index and the middle finger of the left hand. A needle on a 20 ml syringe half filled with normal saline is introduced in one movement at the tip of the left middle finger. The left hand is then lifted from the femoral artery and the needle is carefully withdrawn while gently aspirating on the syringe. The sudden appearance of dark venous blood in the syringe indicates that the needle is correctly positioned. The syringe is carrefully disconnected from the needle and a metallic guide wire advanced down the lumen of the needle and into the vein. The introducer is then put in place as shown in the diagram of plates IX, X, XI, p 33, 36, 37.

Good technique comes with practice. If the position of the needle is inaccurate, it will be withdrawn without having entered the vein. A second attempt may be made but in face of repeated failure, the opposite side should be tried. If the puncture is made too laterally, the femoral artery may be entered, the piston of the syringe recoiling under the pressure of a pulsatile jet of red blood. The needle should be carefully removed and the vessel compressed for a few minutes. Haematoma formation necessitates changing sides. However, several attempts at venous puncture may be made providing dangerous manipulation is avoided. This is usually the result of **lateral movement** of the needle either at the moment of puncture or during withdrawal.

When venous puncture is successful and the vein introducer correctly positioned, a bipolar pacing catheter (USCI C-51) with its end gently curved is advanced into the vein. Its progress should be smooth although there is sometimes a difficulty in navigating the curvature of the lower border of the ilium. Manipulation is monitored by radiological screening as the catheter may form a loop. To and fro movements of the catheter are usually sufficient should the catheter take a false pathway. Looping the catheter in the right atrium sometimes enables the tricuspid valve to be crossed more easily. When correctly positioned in the right ventricle, the catheter assumes an inverse J-shape (Plate XI, p 37). It is important that the catheter tip should be in a **stable position** and this is checked by asking the patient to cough and breath deeply. If all seems satisfactory the pacing threshold should be measured the normal value being below **1 volt and 1 milli-ampere.** It is possible to record a lesion potential by forcing the pacing catheter against the ventricular wall and then, as it is gently withdrawn, it is seen to disappear. The catheter is then connected to an external pacemaker. The amplitude and frequency are set, having firstly checked that the **battery is charged.** The excess wire is looped and placed under the pacemaker box and the whole is strapped to the thigh with a wide adhesive band.

2. Sub-clavicular approach

This technique has the advantage of being quicker and the stability of the pacing catheter is very good. Risk of infection is less than with the femoral approach but the complications of this method are potentially **more serious.** Strict adherence to technique is important.

A needle attached to a half-filled 20 ml syringe of saline is again used. Starting on the left of the patient the angle between the clavicle and the costal cartilage is defined. Lateral movements of the needle permit the operator to guide his way between the two bones and once correctly positioned the same equipment is used as in the previous approach. It is often easier to use a semi-floating pacing catheter as it practically places itself at the apex of the right ventricle, radiological screening permitting a good position within seconds.

3. Brachial approach

The technique involves venous cut down and the risk of displacing the catheter tip by movements of the arm is great. It is therefore unsatisfactory and **should be abandoned.**

Temporary pacing catheters should be left in place for the shortest possible time (24-48 hours) so that complications of infection and displacement of the catheter are minimised. With good technique, the pacing catheter may be left in place for **several days,** providing checks are made of the skin site, threshold of stimulation and of the radiological position of the catheter tip.

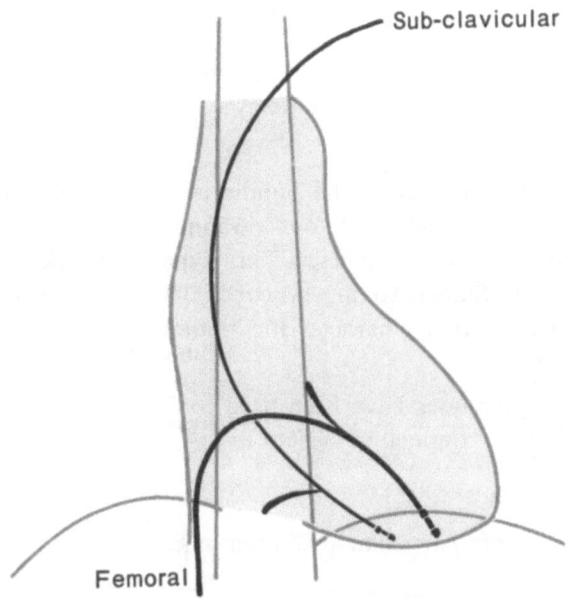

Temporary pacing routes

ELECTROPHYSIOLOGICAL STUDIES

More refined methods have been developed to investigate the problem of potentially fatal syncopes and to determine their association with atrio and intra-ventricular conduction defects. If serious conduction defects are present the anatomical lesion may be localised and the implantation of a pacemaker **considered.**

1. Technique

Electrophysiological studies are to rhythmology what cardiac catheterisation is to valvular heart disease. Using the femoral approach, catheters of the type used for temporary pacing are positioned in the intracardiac cavities under radioscopic surveillance (Plate XII, p 40). Two catheters are usually used: one is advanced to the right ventricle and then gradually withdrawn through the angle of the anterior and septal leaflets of the tricuspid valve. The endocavitary potentials are continually monitored. The catheter is so positioned that the His bundle potential is recorded (Plate XIII, p 41).

The order of deflections observed are:
—The **lower right atrial** potential (A);
—The **His bundle** potential (H) which is quite separate and precedes the first part of the **inter-ventricular septal** depolarisation (V) by **about 40 ms.**

2. Localisation of blocks

Two types of blocks may be recognised by recording the time intervals between the atrial potential and that of the bundle of His and the bundle of His and the start of ventricular depolarisation.

—**Supra-hisian blocks.**

These are usually situated above the bundle of His in the A-V node and are characterised by atrio-hisian delays.

—**Infra-hisian blocks.**

These are usually situated in the bundle of His or its branches and are characterised by a delay of over **55 ms** between His bundle activation and that of its branches. This type of block has a more serious prognosis in Stokes-Adams syncope. Blocks occurring in the bundle of His itself give a characteristic double deflection of the His potential (split His).

The following techniques have been used to exhibit latent conducting blocks by stressing the conduction system.

3. Pharmaco-dynamic studies

These techniques are particularly favored in Europe.

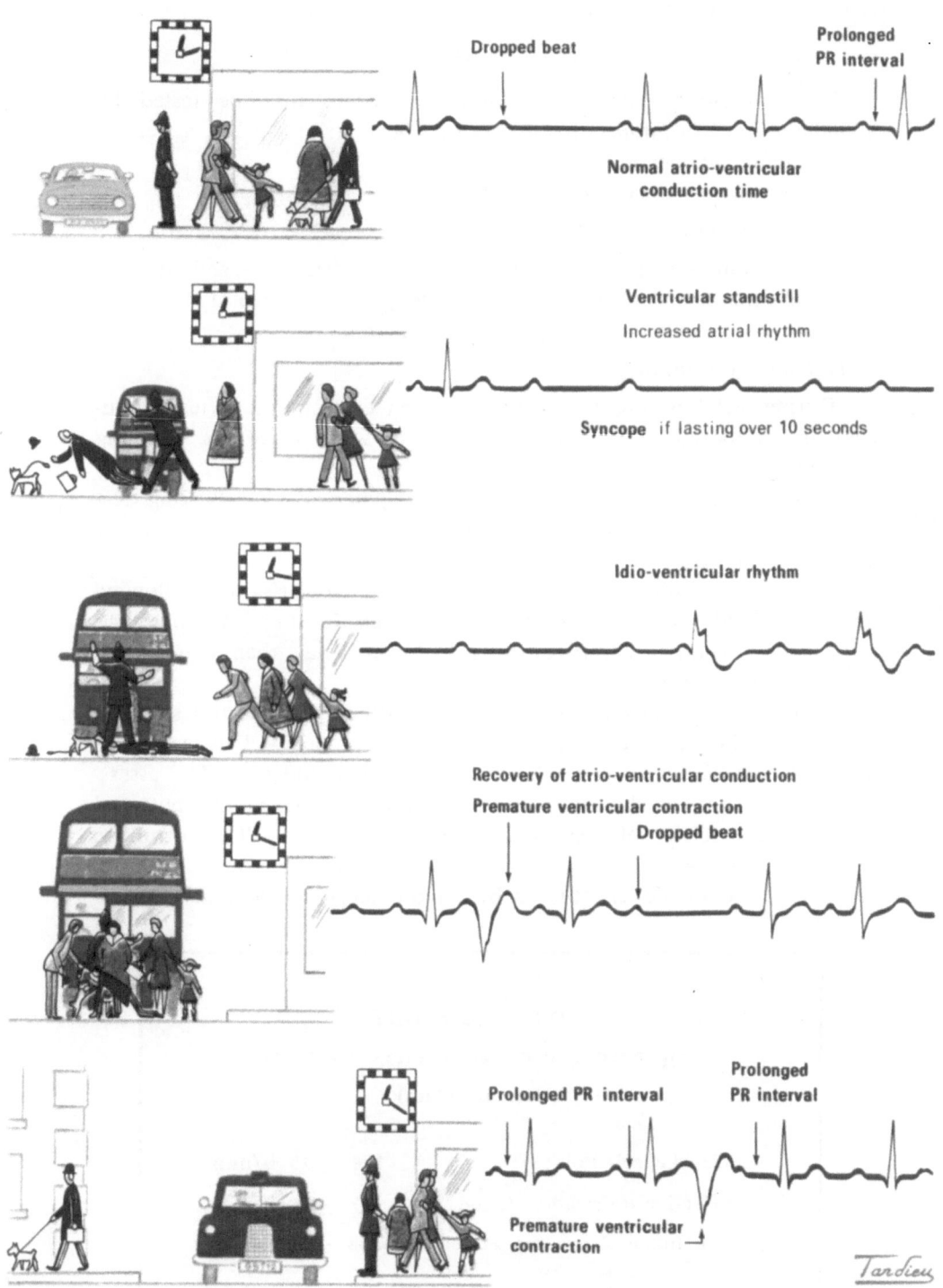

Dropped beat

Prolonged PR interval

Normal atrio-ventricular conduction time

Ventricular standstill

Increased atrial rhythm

Syncope if lasting over 10 seconds

Idio-ventricular rhythm

Recovery of atrio-ventricular conduction

Premature ventricular contraction

Dropped beat

Prolonged PR interval

Prolonged PR interval

Premature ventricular contraction

Tardieu

Simultaneous injection of substances like Procainamide or **Ajmaline** which depress A-V conduction may prolong the H-V interval and so suggest a latent conduction defect.

4. Endocavitary stimulation studies (Plate XIV, p 45)

The integrity of the A-V conduction system may be tested by stimulation of the upper point of the right atrium using a second endocavitary catheter.

There are two ways of doing this:

—*The Wenkebach point*

The atrium is stimulated at a progressively faster rate and the rate at which the atrial tachycardia is **no longer conducted** 1/1 to the ventricle is recorded (normally at 174 ± 15/min).

—*Test stimulus technique*

During atrial pacing (drive stimulus) an extrastimulus (test stimulus) is interposed every 8-10 driven beats with a **varying coupling interval.**

● If the coupling interval is long, depolarisation following test stimulus will be conducted to the ventricle with an **identical time** delay to that of the drive stimuli rhythm.

● If the coupling interval is shortened, depolarisation following the test stimulus will be progressively **slowed in the A-V node** and ventricular response will occur after a longer delay than that of the drive stimuli rhythm.

● If the coupling interval is shortened still further the test stimulus will be **blocked** as the refractory period is attained. This occurs at about 290 ms for a basal rhythm of between 600-700 ms. The assessment of H-V interval by the catheter recording the His bundle potential enables the precision of a supra- or infra-hisian blocks. This technique often produces results when the rest of investigation has been negative, as the A-V conduction is studied by a more sensitive method.

DYNAMIC STUDY

OF THE A-V CONDUCTION SYSTEM

(Normal values)

Wenckebach Point	174 ± 15 b/min
Effective Refractory Period	297 ± 20 ms
Functional Refractory Period	388 ± 39 ms

1- Defibrillator **1'-** Electrodes **2-** Electrode gel **3-** Triple channel ECG **4-** Isoprenaline **5-** Sodium bicarbonate
6- ECG monitor

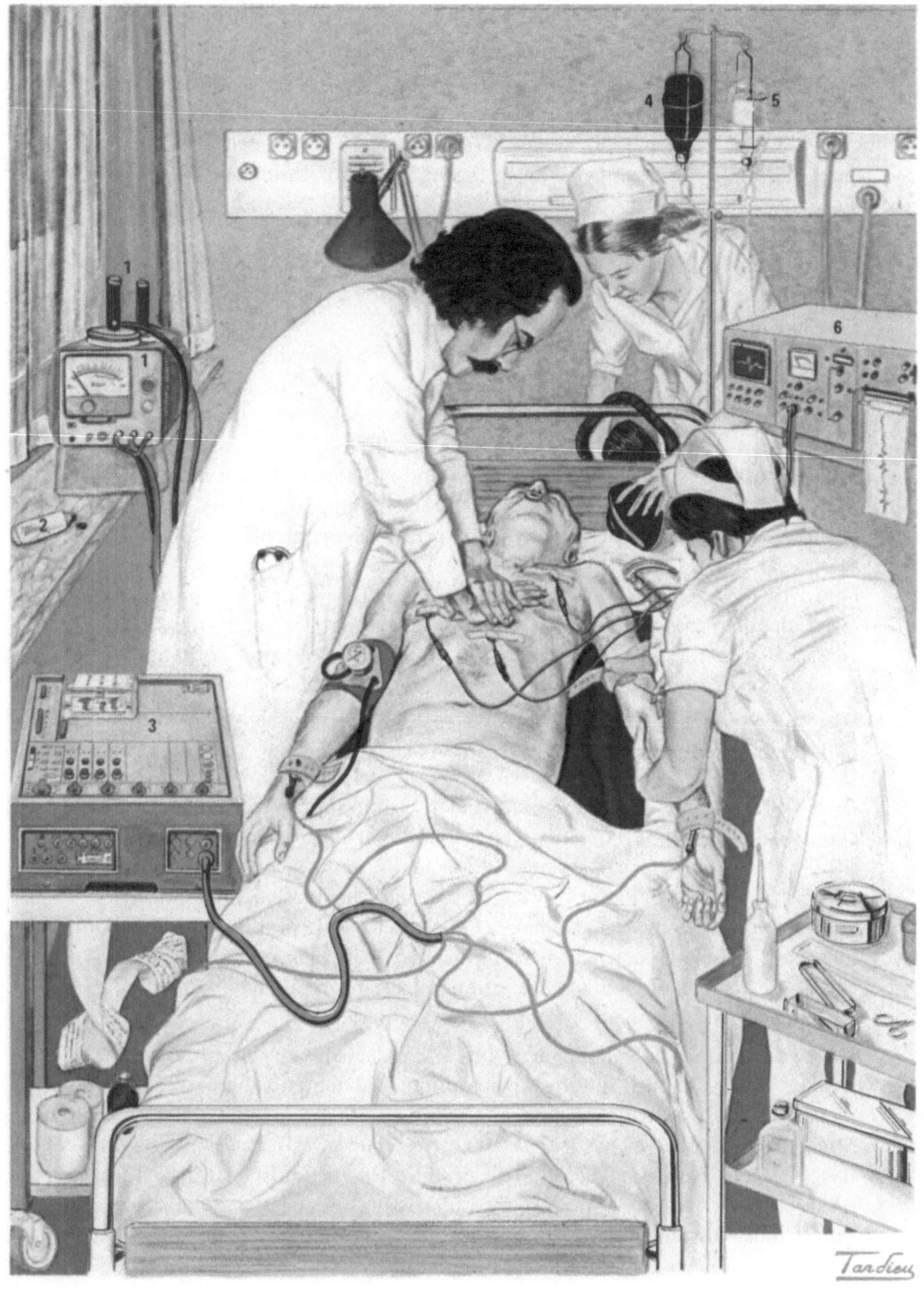

THE USE OF PACEMAKERS
IN DISEASES OTHER THAN A-V BLOCK

The success of pacing in the treatment of the bradycardia of complete heart block has led to its use in patients with periodic episodes of **bradycardia** unrelated to conduction defects. Recent advances in our knowledge of endocavitary electrocardiology have resulted in the use of temporary and permanent pacing in the treatment of certain **tachycardias.**

1. Sino-atrial block and sinus bradycardia

Sino-atrial block is the result of either a fault in production of activation or in its transmission to the atria or a combination of both. The ECG shows a periodic absence of the "P" wave with absence of ventricular depolarisation. In some cases, a considerable delay in sinus activity may be recorded with irregular "P" waves. The clinical picture is of a vagal syndrome with bradycardia, hypotension, tiredness, and frequent syncopal episodes. Diagnosis is often difficult as the ECG may be normal especially after exertion and emotion. Taped monitoring (Holter monitoring, Plate XXII, p 65) is in these cases the principal means of diagnosis. Electrophysiological studies are of limited value as sinusal function tests give appreciable false negative results. Pacing improves these patients. When ventricular pacing is used, a retrograde atrial depolarisation might be obtained, so the pacemaker has to be adjusted at a rate of 60/min. just to take over for more pronounced bradycardia. Atrial pacing is the method of choice in these cases but the A-V conduction must first be checked by electrophysiological studies.

2. Bradycardia-tachycardia syndrome

This syndrome is usually associated with supra-ventricular tachycardias alternating atrial extrasystoles and periods of atrial flutter or fibrillation. These are suddenly followed by an iso-electric interval of several seconds until sinus rhythm is re-established, often after an atrioventricular junctional escape beat. The alternation of bradycardia and tachycardia is characteristic of this syndrome. The periods of tachycardia or tachy-arrhythmias are often experienced as palpitations and the sinusal pause as near syncope by these patients.

Medical treatment of this arrhythmia is unsatisfactory as drugs which depress the excitability of the myocardium also tend to increase sinusal blocks and drugs which increase the automaticity of the sinus node often predispose to tachycardias. The association of a **pacemaker with drugs** which depress myocardial excitability is the most effective form of treatment. Atrial stimulation would seem the best way of pacing but it must be remembered that many of these patients also have A-V conduction defects and so bifocal stimulation would be the ideal method.

Pl. VIII

DEFIBRILLATION 1-Battery powered oscilloscope and defibrillator 2- Electrode gel 3- Defibrillator button 4- Defibrillator paddles 5- ECG electrodes connected to needles introduced under the skin

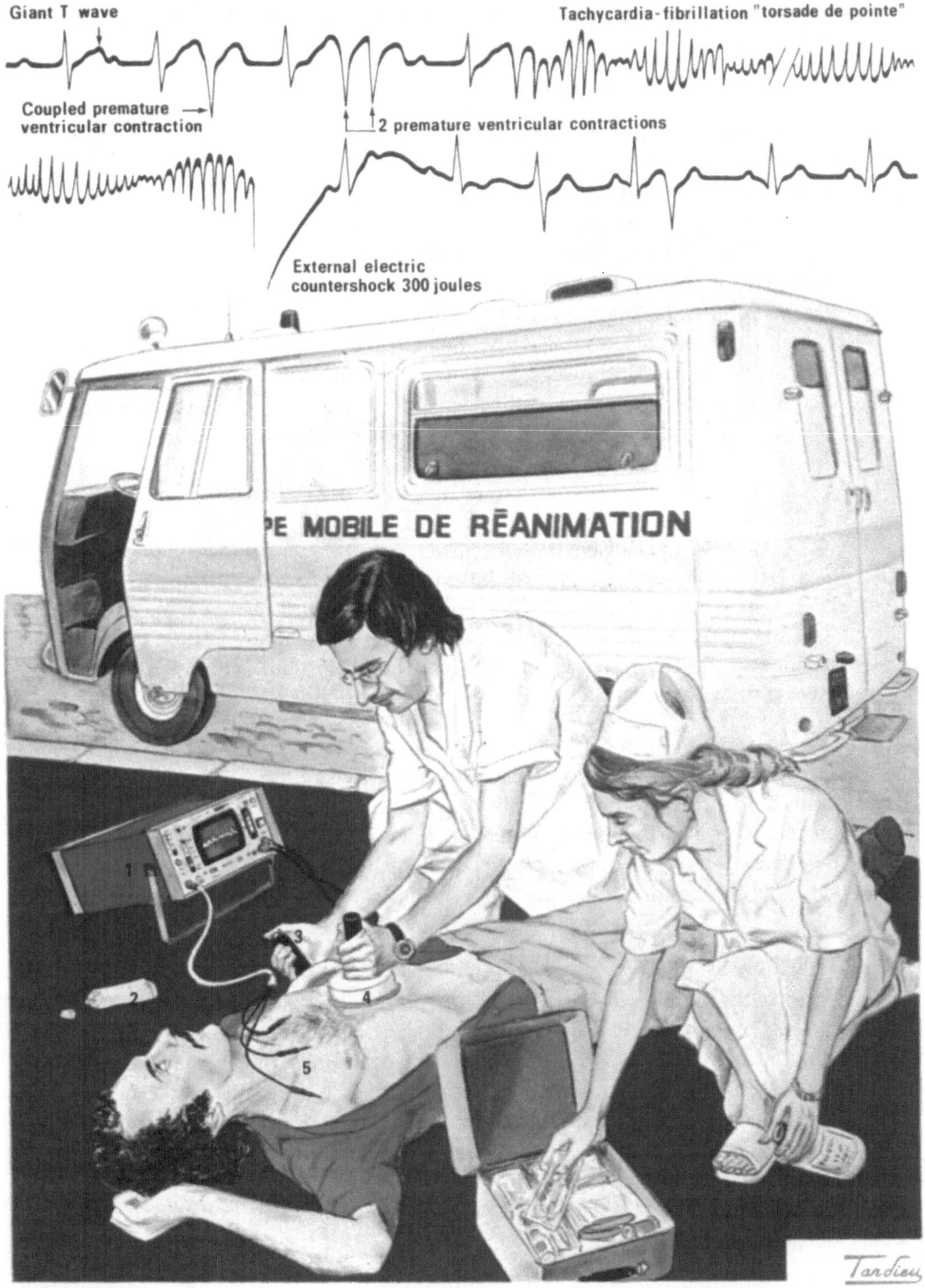

Giant T wave

Tachycardia-fibrillation "torsade de pointe"

Coupled premature ventricular contraction

2 premature ventricular contractions

External electric countershock 300 joules

PE MOBILE DE RÉANIMATION

Tardieu

There is a high incidence of systemic embolism in this syndrome (at the time of reestablishment of sinus rhythm). Anticoagulants should therefore be prescribed to all patient who have no clear contra-indications.

3. Pacing in tachycardias

Experience gained by the use of temporary pacing in intensive care units and the success of intracardiac electrical studies have rapidly increased our knowledge of the mode of production of many arrhythmias. Pacing techniques perfected during these investigations or study of the ECG characteristics of the arrhythmia have opened the way to treatment of certain cases of tachycardia by normal or specially adapted pacemakers. The main uses of the pacemakers according to the individual case are (1) to pace the heart at a minimal rhythm so that myocardial depressing drugs may be prescribed at sufficient doses, (2) to stop the attacks of tachycardia as they occur, either automatically or manually, (3) to prevent recurrence of tachycardia by permanent pacing at a fast enough rate.

—Ventricular tachycardia

An attack of ventricular tachycardia may be **stopped** by one or two correctly timed ventricular extra-stimuli or by a burst or rapid stimuli triggered by the patient with the use of a magnet placed on top of the pacemaker. **Prevention** of ventricular tachycardia is sometimes possible by pacing at a rate faster than the basal rhythm, but slower than the tachycardia. Atrial stimulation is the method of choice.

—Atrial and junctional tachycardias

These arrhythmias may also be managed by pacing. A device which sends one or two stimuli a calculated coupling interval or, depending on the case, an atrial stimulation just after normal atrial activation may be used. The prevention of junctional tachycardias may sometimes be achieved by continual pacing at a faster rate than the basal rhythm.

—Wolff-Parkinson-White syndrome

This was the first disease in which a pacemaker was used to stop paroxystic tachycardia. A burst of stimuli may be triggered by the placing of a magnet next to the pacemaker (so as to compete with the abnormal rhythm). One stimulation will eventually fall in the sensitive time zone and so block the tachycardia. A **radio-frequency receiver** may also be used in association with a regulated external transmitter. **Prevention** of tachycardia in the WPW syndrome may also be achieved. Pacing would appear to be an intermediate form of management between drug therapy and surgery where the latter may be considered too dangerous.

In contrast to the treatment of A-V blocks, the treatment of tachy-cardias by pacing requires considerable attention to the rate of pacing, the site of stimulation, etc. Each parameter must be adjusted for **every single case.** The use of a pacemaker is only indicated when one is certain that anti-arrhythmic treatment is ineffective after rigorous and often repeated electrophysiological studies.

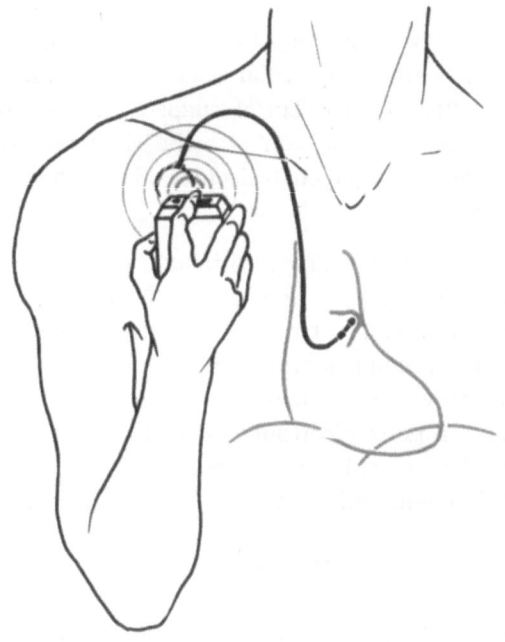

Termination of supra-ventricular tachycardia
by radio-frequency pacemaker

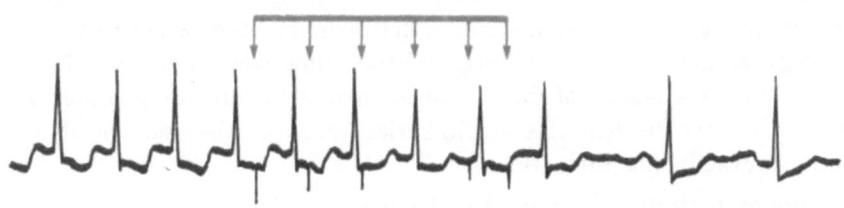

PACEMAKERS AND THEIR FUNCTION

A) TYPES OF PACING

In unipolar stimulation one cardiac electrode is used, the other being either the metal casing or one of the sides of the pacemaker. The cardiac electrode is always **negative** as it gives the lowest threshold, that is to say the weakest stimulus to start ventricular depolarisation.

2. Endocavitary and epicardial

Electrodes may be positioned in the myocardium itself. Of this type the Chardack epicardo-myocardial electrode is the most often used (Plate XV, p 49). It is a spiral shaped piece of platinum which is inserted through a small incision into the right or left ventricular wall. The electrode has an L-shaped trajectory, the second part being parallel to the epicardium.

Endocavitary catheters are positioned, using the venous approach, at the apex of the right ventricle or on the floor of the right ventricle in the paratricuspid area. Unipolar electrodes are cylindrical and are connected to the pacemaker electrode by an isolated spiral wire. Most transilastic electrodes have a widened end to facilitate contact and stability at the apex. Bipolar electrodes differ from the unipolar type in that a second ring-shaped pole is present 1·5 to 3 cms from the other electrode. It is connected to a second isolated wire (Plate I, p 9).

B) THE PACEMAKER

The main components are an energy source and an electronic circuit.

1. Energy source

The most frequently used energy source in the past has been **mercury batteries** (which have a life span of 2·5 to 4 years). 4 or 5 batteries are needed, connected in series, to produce enough current. The batteries are not sealed as an alkaline electrolyte is used which gives off hydrogen as the batteries discharge. When they run down, the electric charge falls in a matter of days, a phenomenon luckily compensated for by the fact that the batteries are in series, and that they do not all run down at exactly the same time.

Lithium batteries have now completely replaced mercury power source. They have the advantage of being more compact, hermetically sealed and have a life span of 5-10 years with a steady rate of discharge so that replacement may be planned ahead.

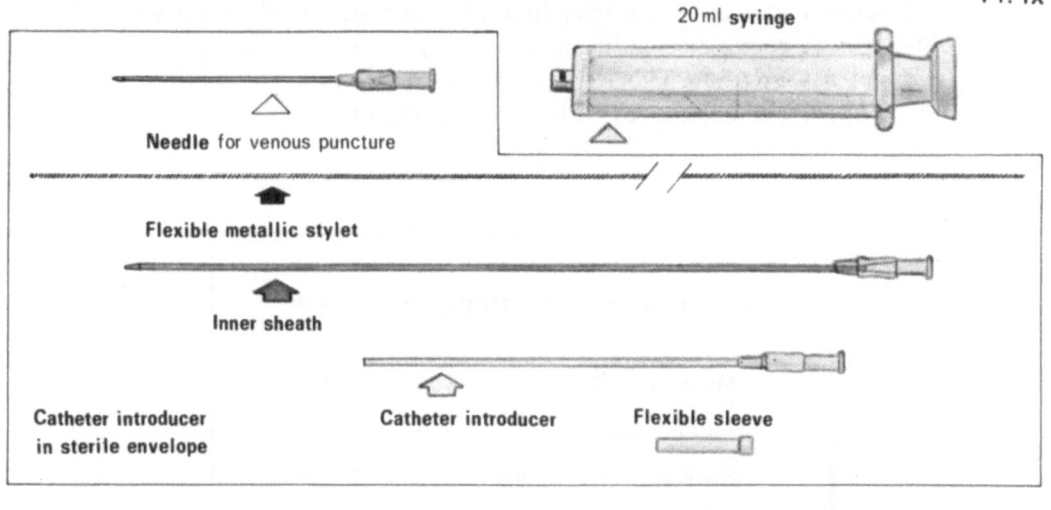

20 ml **syringe**

Needle for venous puncture

Flexible metallic stylet

Inner sheath

**Catheter introducer
in sterile envelope**

Catheter introducer

Flexible sleeve

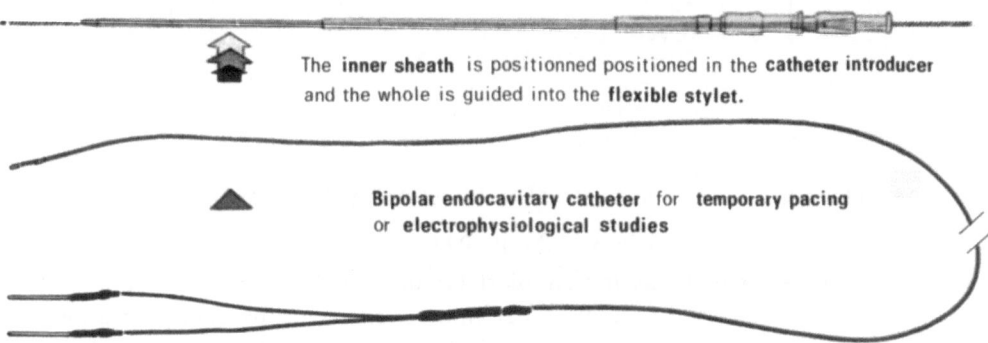

The **inner sheath** is positionned positioned in the **catheter introducer** and the whole is guided into the **flexible stylet**.

Bipolar endocavitary catheter for temporary pacing or **electrophysiological studies**

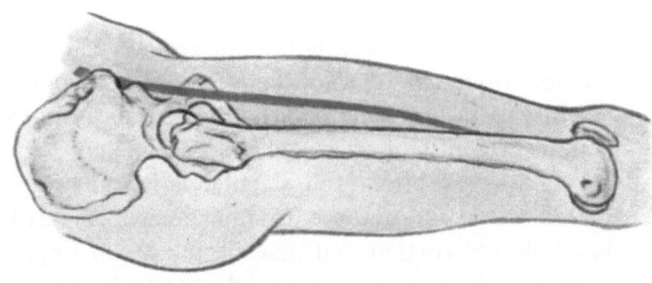

Anatomical relationships
of the femoral vein.

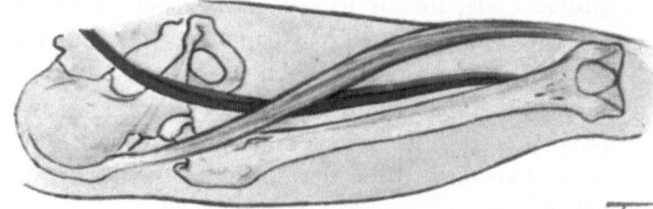

Tardieu

33

Nuclear batteries have a very long life span and would seem ideally suited for a young person in need of a pacemaker. However, they represent a source of radio-activity which creates problems of its own, not the least administrative. Their use is therefore limited.

TYPICAL PACEMAKERS LIFE TIME

Mercury Cells	2 to 4 years
Lithium Cells	5 to 10 years
Nuclear Power Source	> 10 years

---

2. Basic electronic circuits

The function of the pacemaker is determined by this element:

—*A fixed rate unit* (Plate XX, p 61)

This pacemaker has the simplest circuit which transforms the continuous current into 70 impulses per minute of 1-2 milliseconds duration. Its advantages are the simplicity of the circuit and the fact that little current is used up (most of the energy available is used in stimulating the myocardium rather than running the circuit itself). They are relatively cheap and very reliable.

The main drawback is the appearance of **competitive rhythms** (interference rhythms) if A-V conduction is spontaneously re-established. When this occurs some ventricular depolarisations are produced by the sinusal rhythm and others by the pacemaker. The number of responses are limited as after each depolarisation the heart enters a refractory period. The interference rhythm creates an artificial extrasystole in a basal sinusal rhythm and may be felt as an unpleasant sensation by the patient. If an electrical stimulus falls in the vulnerable zone of the cardiac cycle, that is to say at the **peak of the T-wave,** about 140 ms after the spontaneous QRS complex, ventricular fibrillation may occur. This is a real problem in patients with acute myocardial ischaemia, but there is a little risk in a "normal" heart. However, a patient with a pacemaker is not protected from coronary artery disease. Therefore, pacemakers have been developed to avoid this problem, demand pacemakers.

—QRS inhibited demand pacemakers (QRS —)

These devices are equiped with a **sensing circuit** in addition to the pacing circuit so' as to detect the autonomous electrical activity of the heart (Plate XIX, p 59). Potentials of the order of 10 mV which occur during spontaneous cardiac depolarisations are picked up by the pacemaker electrodes. These potentials, after amplification, block the pacing circuit for a certain period of time so creating a definite pacemaker pacing interval. When this time has elapsed without detection of further spontaneous electrical activity, the pacing circuit discharges an electrical stimulus. On the other hand if spontaneous activity is detected the pacing circuit is re-inhibited and another stimulus may only be triggered after the regulated time interval has elapsed. Accordingly, a pacing stimulus will always fall at one pacing interval after any spontaneous QRS complex and therefore will never fall in the dangerous zone which occurs as previously explained, at the peak of the T-wave, and lasts about 40 ms.

When there is no spontaneous activity, the demand pacemaker paces continually and cannot be distinguished from a fixed rate pacemaker from the surface ECG tracing. If the patient has a spontaneous rhythm faster than that of the pacemaker the pacemaker will be permanently inhibited. Under these conditions it is impossible to determine form the ECG whether or not the patient has a pacemaker without further tests.

—QRS triggered demand pacemakers (QRS+)

This type of pacemaker also has an electronic system of taking command if the spontaneous cardiac activity falls below the basal rhythm of the sensing circuit. However if the spontaneous rhythm is faster than that of the pacemaker, a pacing stimulus will be seen **inside the QRS complex,** that is to say in the absolute refractory period, instead of complete absence of pacing activity as seen with QRS inhibited pacemakers (Plate XX, p 61). The ECG is often more difficult to read. The main advantage of this set up is that it is possible to accelerate the pacemaker rhythm by external means. Electrical impulses are passed across the surface of the thorax using ECG leads. These currents are too weak to stimulate the heart but the pacemaker interprets them as QRS complexes and so triggers a stimulus, pacing the heart if it falls outside the refractory period. In any case the faster external rate takes command sooner or later. This is a useful property when treating some cases of heart failure or arrhythmias.

—Atrial synchronous pacing

Atrial synchronous stimulation is the most physiological method as

(The same technique is used either for **temporary pacing** or **electrophysiological investigations**)

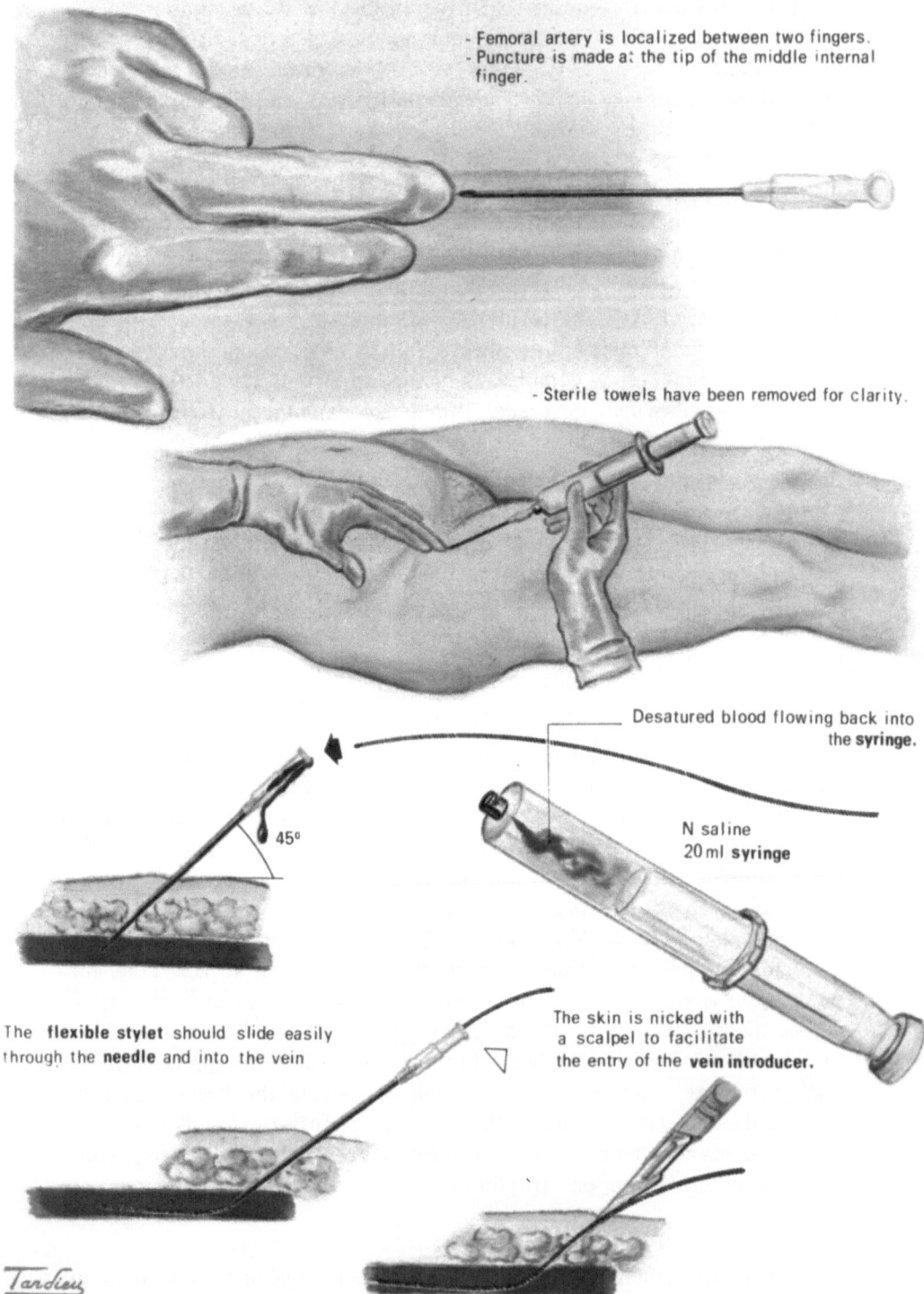

- Femoral artery is localized between two fingers.
- Puncture is made at the tip of the middle internal finger.

- Sterile towels have been removed for clarity.

Desatured blood flowing back into the **syringe.**

N saline
20 ml **syringe**

The **flexible stylet** should slide easily through the **needle** and into the vein

The skin is nicked with a scalpel to facilitate the entry of the **vein introducer.**

45°

Tardieu

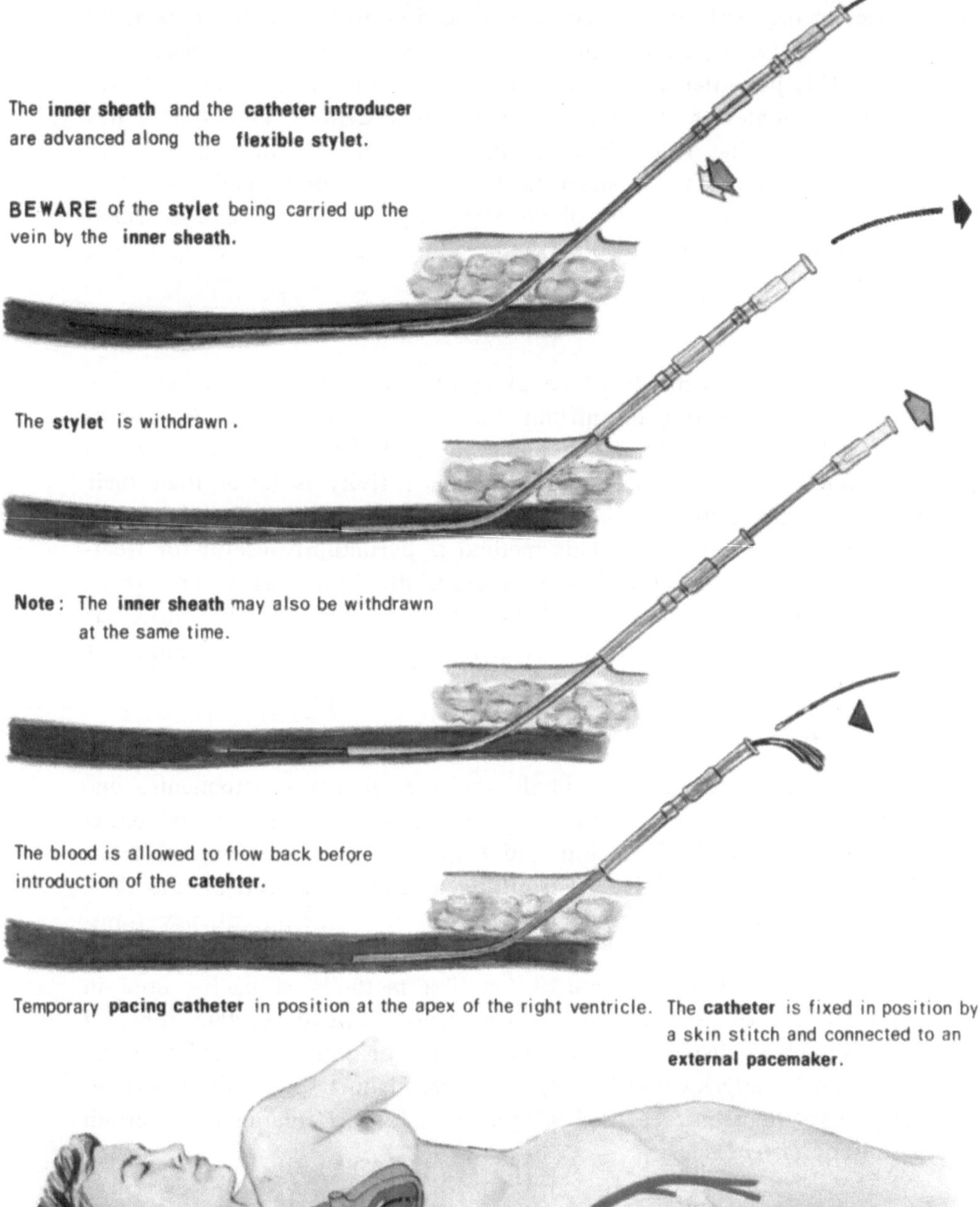

The **inner sheath** and the **catheter introducer**
are advanced along the **flexible stylet**.

BEWARE of the **stylet** being carried up the
vein by the **inner sheath**.

The **stylet** is withdrawn.

Note : The **inner sheath** may also be withdrawn
       at the same time.

The blood is allowed to flow back before
introduction of the **catehter**.

Temporary **pacing catheter** in position at the apex of the right ventricle. The **catheter** is fixed in position by
a skin stitch and connected to an
external pacemaker.

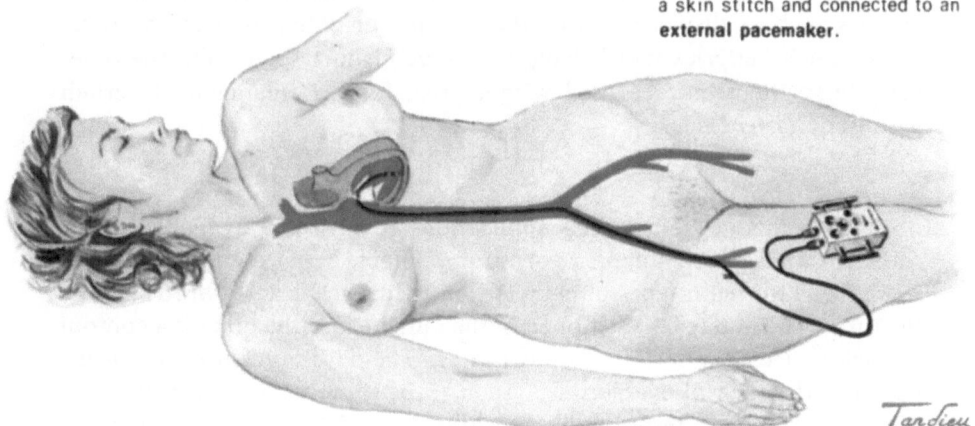

37

ventricular depolarisation is regulated according to the spontaneous atrial activity. Atrial depolarisation is detected by a specially designed electrode. This potential triggers a ventricular stimulus after a time interval that **approximates the normal atrio-ventricular delay.** This system has the advantage that it produces a higher cardiac output and a better effort tolerance which is particularly useful in young patients. The disadvantage is the necessity of an extra atrial sensing electrode which is often difficult to position whether the endocardial or epicardial approach is used.

—Bifocal pacing

Bifocal pacing consists of coupling two command pacemakers side by side one stimulating the atrium, the other the ventricle. An appropriate delay is built into the system. Each of the demand pacemakers is inhibited if the spontaneous ventricular activity is faster than their basic rate and only functions when the spontaneous rhythm of the respective structures fails. This method is particularly useful for treating patients with atrial arrhythmias especially bradycardias and those who, in addition to sinus node failure, have associated atrio-ventricular conduction defects. Bifocal pacemakers necessitate the positionning of two endocavitary electrodes.

—Radio-frequency pacing

This method of pacing entails the use of two components, one internal and the other external. A small **receiver** (there are no batteries) is placed under the skin and connected to the pacing catheter. When necessary, a reel-like transmitting antenna is placed on the skin, covering the receiving capsule and relayed to a radio-frequency transmitter. The transmitter may be programmed to the needs of the individual patient. This was one of the first methods of pacing used in the treatment of A-V blocks. There were however certain inherent dangers such as displacement of the antenna or exhaustion of the radio transmitter's batteries which have a relatively short span. On the other hand this system may be used without risk for the treatment of certain **paraxystic arrhythmias.**

—Atrial pacing

This technique had limited applications because the available pacing catheters were poorly adapted for atrial contact, better equipment is now available. Two main types of catheter are used: One is a J-shaped catheter the tip of which may be positioned in the auricle, and the other is a contour shaped catheter for coronary sinus pacing. The development of new atrial pacing catheters will enable this system to be more widely used. Its main advantage is that it respects the physiological A-V conduction in patients

1 - Ink jet recorder.
2 - Programmed pacemaker.
3 - Oscilloscope.
4 - ECG monitoring
5 - X Ray equipment.
6 - Video monitor.

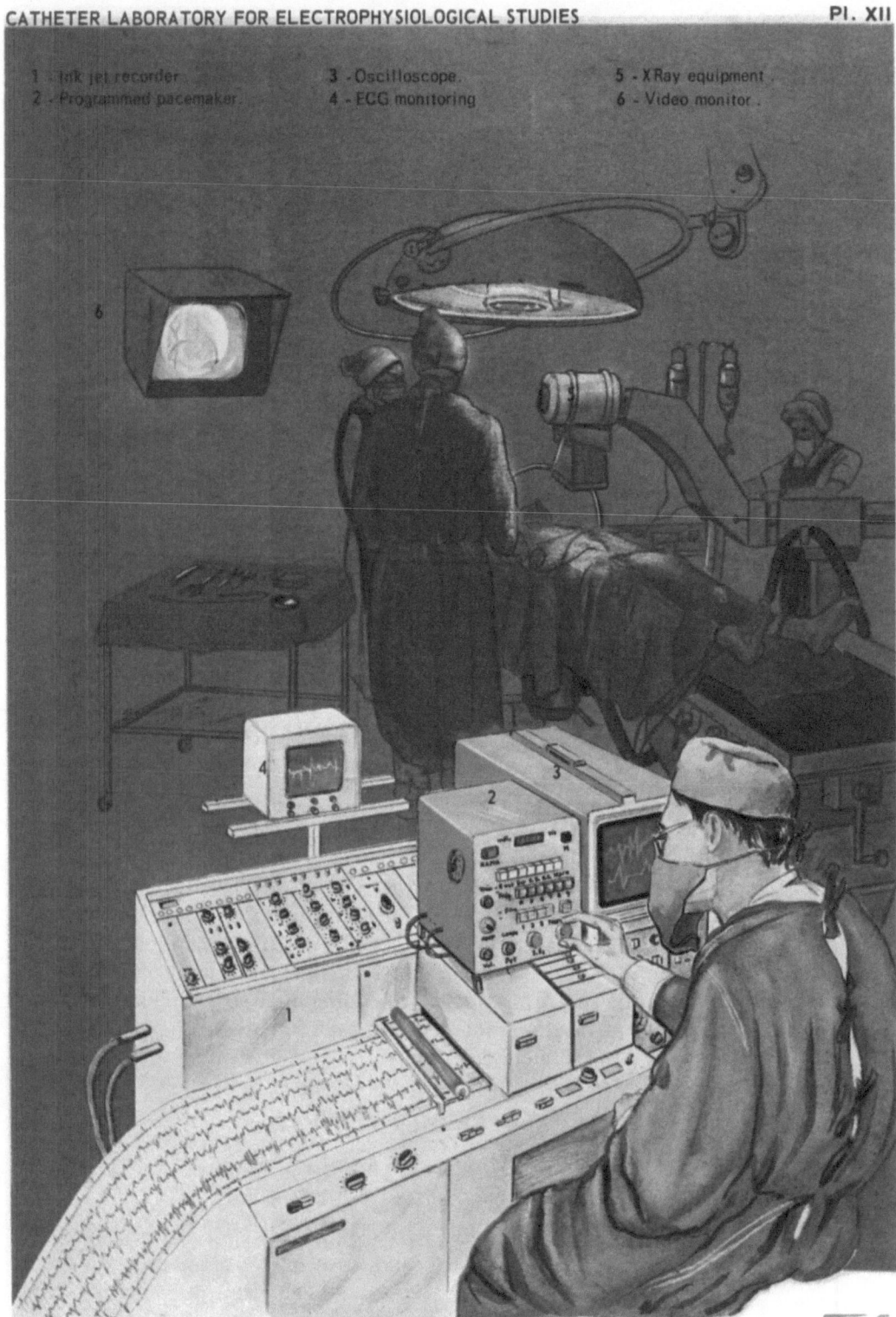

without A-V block. Its main indications are the treatment of sino-atrial block bradycardia-tachycardia syndrome (where a bifocal pacing method may be used), and in the prevention or treatment of some arrhythmias.

3. New systems

—Programmable pacemakers

The function of these pacemakers may be adjusted from patient to patient. For example, a rhythm of 70/min may be too fast for a patient who had long periods of complete heart block before the implantation of his pacemaker. On the other hand, in patients with "Torsades de pointes" the rhythm may be too slow. Also in patients in whom the pacing catheter is well positioned with a low threshold of around 1 volt, there is no point in stimulating with a potential of 5 or 6 volts. In these cases, it is useful to be able to reduce the amplitude or duration of stimulation whilst allowing sufficient margin for safety so that the life of pacemaker batteries may be preserved.

This is the reason why manufacturers have developed pacemakers which may be programmed externally. Depending on the actual model used a rotating magnetic field is placed against the pacemaker. This attracts a small magnet situated in a sealed compartment of the pacemaker. Its rotation alters the setting of the pacemaker potentiometer. In other models electro-magnetic impulses transmitted through the skin to a magnetic switch are relayed to an electronic circuit which decodes the number of impulses. A number of electronic switches then adjust the electrical resistance to the programed value.

—Vario-pacemaker

This device allows the **threshold level** to be measured in a non-invasive way. A specially designed internal circuit is triggered by the use of a magnet. The following pacemaker functions result: 1) a fixed rate, 2) increase in frequency of stimulation from 70 to 100/min (in recent models a constant amplitude is achieved during the first 15 consecutive impulses), 3) then during the following 15 impulses the amplitude of stimulation decreased uniformly. If the amplitude between each impulse is known the threshold level may be accurately determined.

ELECTRIC PACEMAKER FEATURES		
	TYPICAL	EXHAUSTED
Voltage	5-6 V	<3 V
Current	10 mA	<5 mA
Pulse width	0·8 ms	>1·2 ms
Period	857 ms (70 b/mn)	998 ms (60 b/min)
QRS sensitivity	2 mV	>3 mV

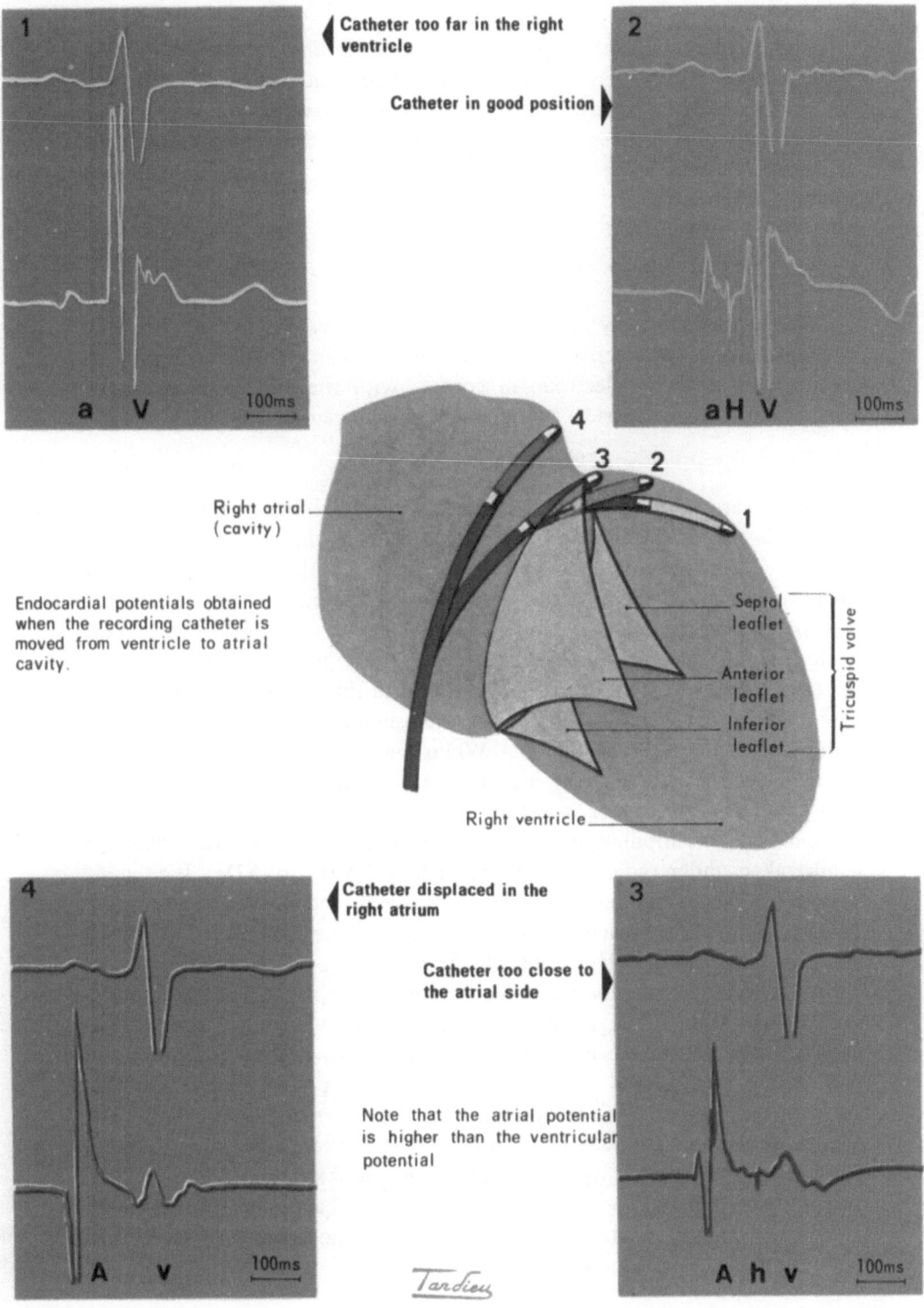

Catheter too far in the right ventricle

Catheter in good position

Right atrial (cavity)

Endocardial potentials obtained when the recording catheter is moved from ventricle to atrial cavity.

Septal leaflet

Anterior leaflet

Inferior leaflet

Tricuspid valve

Right ventricle

Catheter displaced in the right atrium

Catheter too close to the atrial side

Note that the atrial potential is higher than the ventricular potential

Tardieu

IMPLANTATION OF PACEMAKERS

The implantation of a pacemaker involves the introduction of a foreign body made of metal, synthetic rubber and artificial resin into the human body. Bacterial contamination may have serious and potentially fatal consequences so that it is essential that the operation is undertaken under **strict aseptic conditions** (Plate XVI, p 51) and as **quickly** as possible.

A) ENDOCARDIAL PACING

The most frequently used method (95 % cases) is the implantation of a pacemaker connected to an endocavitary catheter. The aim is to position the catheter electrode in contact with the endocardium of the apex of the right ventricle using a peripheral venous approach.

1. Venous approaches (Plate XVII, p 55)

There are several venous approaches possible but the one usually chosen is the **right cephalic** using an incision in the delto-pectoral skin crease. If the vein is found to be usable the catheter and pacemaker may be implanted through the one incision. A pocket is prepared for the pacemaker anterior to the pectoralis major. If the cephalic vein is too narrow, tortuous or thrombosed a second incision is made at the level of the right external jugular vein, two to three fingerbreadths above the clavicle. In some cases, the anterior jugular veins are used and in others, even the internal jugular. When the pacemaker and catheter are introduced through different incisions, a subcutaneous tunnel has to be effected from the site of insertion of the catheter to the pocket of the pacemaker. Manipulation of the catheter in the veins and heart is undertaken under radioscopic control (Plate XVIII, p 57). It is made easier by a stylet, the end of which is gently curved in order to facilitate the crossing of the tricuspid valve. The catheter is advanced to the **outflow tract** of the right ventricle or the pulmonary infundibulum in order to avoid a false pathway in the coronary sinus or posterior interventricular vein. The catheter is then withdrawn with the stylet in place. This causes the catheter to slide over the wall of the heart and fall to the floor of the right ventricle. Its end projects **under** the shadow of the cupola of the left diaphragm when correctly positioned. The catheter must never be pushed forward with the guide wire in place as it may perforate the right ventricle. The catheter should be **immobile** during spontaneous or paced ventricular contractions. To and fro movements in the ventricle and perpendicular movements of more than 0·5 cm must be prevented.

2. Measuring the threshold

When the radiological position is satisfactory the thresholds are measured. Using a calibrated adjustable external pacemaker, the strength of stimulation is gradually decreased until there is **no ventricular response**. The threshold should be less than 1 volt or 1 milli-ampere. When this is not so, the catheter is moved slightly to a site of better activation. When the threshold is acceptable, the catheter is firmly fixed in the vein with two non-resorbable sutures.

> **TYPICAL ACUTE THRESHOLDS**
>
> Voltage   0·6 ±0·3 V
>
> Current   0·7 ±0·4 mA

3. Implanting the pacemaker

The pacemaker box is connected to the catheter and implanted between the pectoralis major and the skin after having **checked** that the connection is sound and watertight. The function of the pacemaker is checked, either for spontaneous activity or with the use of a magnet. In thin patients, the pacemaker can be pushed through the pectoralis major and positioned posteriorly. The first technique leads to more frequent cutaneous reactions while the second is associated with a higher incidence of post-operative haematoma and migration of the pacemaker box to the axillary regions. If there has been a substantial blood loss during the operation or if the patient is taking anti-coagulants, it is necessary to put in a redon drain for 24-48 hours.

4. Post-operative period

In practically all cases, the post-operative period is uncomplicated. The patient is kept in bed for the first 4 days to prevent early displacement of the catheter. A slight temperature may be observed during this period but should disappear after 5-6 days. The skin sutures are removed on the 7th or 8th day, and the patient is allowed home between the 10th and the 14th day. The discomfort felt on moving the arm usually disappears in the first two weeks. Excessive washing over the pacemaker site should be avoided for a short while. The patient usually returns to normal activity within a few days or weeks of convalescence.

5. Early complications

After implantation a reaction to the **foreign body** occurs around the electrodes with oedema and local inflammation. This will separate the electrode from the excitable endocardium causing a **normal increase** in the threshold from 1 to 2 volts (potential of the pacemaker is 4 to 5 volts). The threshold then gradually returns to almost its original value. In some patients, an **abnormal elevation** of the threshold value may be observed. If the catheter is pressed too strongly against the ventricular wall, it will tend to go through it by separating the myocardial fibres. In other patients the catheter may progressively withdraw into the ventricular cavity. These minimal displacements are not usually apparent on X-ray. Whatever the cause, the threshold value increases and risks becoming greater than the amplitude of stimulation leading to exit block at first **intermittent** and then permanent. This fault is often preceeded by a defect in the **sensing system** of demand pacemakers. Gross early **displacements** of the catheter electrode may be observed on X-ray. The catheter may be observed in the pulmonary infundibulum, atrium or even inferior vena cava. These incidents are relatively rare (5 %) nowadays as the quality of the equipment has improved and the **skill of the operator** increased with experience. In the early days of pacing this problem led to symptoms as serious as syncope, but now most patients are operated on at the paroxistic stage of A-V block and pacemaker failure is detected by using the magnet test in the first few days after implantation. In repositioning the catheter electrode, the same technique is used as before. Repeated operations are **painful** and require a deep level of anaesthesia. The same aseptic precautions must be taken.

B) DIRECT MYOCARDIAL PACING

This method of pacing is much less frequently employed (5 % of cases). The surgery required is much more complicated (Plate XV, p 49). Either a thoracotomy or an epigastric approach is used under general anaesthetic and assisted respiration.

1. Positioning of the electrodes

The parietal pericardium is exposed though a skin incision in the subxiphoid zone. A retractor is used to keep the incision open and to lift the sternum. The parietal pericardium is incised to expose the apex of the heart and the right heart margin. The electrodes are inserted into the myocardium, a delicate manoeuvre when the heart is beating spontaneously. If the heart is being temporarily paced, a brief period of rapid stimulation followed by stopping the pacing will stop the heart and make the positioning of the electrodes easier.

2. Checking the threshold

This is carried out under identical conditions to those already outlined. The threshold should be measured for each electrode and the one with the lower value will be connected to the **negative pole** (bipolar stimulation).

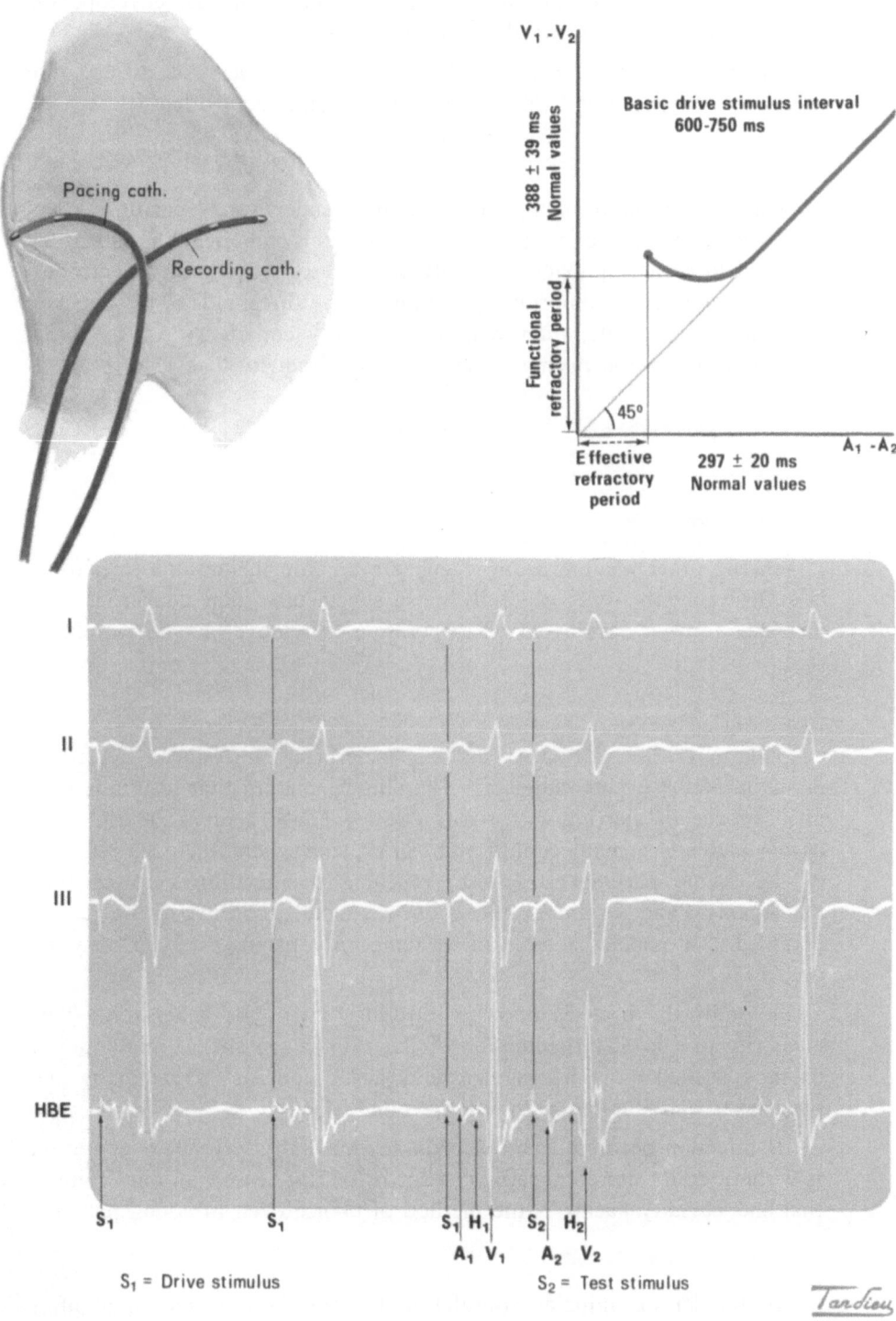

$V_1 - V_2$

388 ± 39 ms
Normal values

Basic drive stimulus interval
600-750 ms

Functional refractory period

45°

Effective refractory period

297 ± 20 ms
Normal values

$A_1 - A_2$

Pacing cath.

Recording cath.

I

II

III

HBE

S_1 S_1 S_1 H_1 S_2 H_2
                         A_1 V_1 A_2 V_2

S_1 = Drive stimulus S_2 = Test stimulus

Tardieu

45

3. Implanting the pacemaker

This is carried out in the sub-xiphoïd area or in the envelope of the rectus abdominis, using the same incision.

The. advantages of this technique are that it does not expose the operator to radiation and there is no early displacement of the electrode.

4. Post-operative period

This is often more of a problem than in endocavitary pacing. Post-pericardectomy syndrome is the most frequent complication and it is observed to a varying extent in 30-40 % of cases. Epicardial electrodes are not exempt from abnormal elevations of the threshold. This appears much later, as a rule, than with endocavitary catheters. In the long term ruptures of the pacing wires are more frequent.

C) COMPLICATIONS INDEPENDENT OF THE METHOD OF IMPLANTATION

1. Hematoma

Among other complications which are all rare, hematoma formation is quite frequent. It is generally more spectacular than dangerous and disappears in ten days or so. Re-operation to remove clots is extremely rare.

2. Infection

This may arise in two ways: The bacteria are introduced by contamination of the pacing catheter. The clinical picture that results is that of a septicaemia starting with rigors and leading to a rapid deterioration of the patient's general conditions. The management includes **removal of the whole pacemaker system,** repeated haemocultures to identify the organism and a rational antibiotic treatment according to the results obtained. If pacing is essential a temporary pacing catheter may be used.

Secondly the bacteria may be introduced with the generator. This gives rise to a local inflammation of the skin at the site of implantation of the pacemaker. The management again consists of removing the pacemaker and **implanting it on the other side.**

If infection occurs on an epicardio-myocardial electrode, re-operation is without doubt more **dangerous** and it is for this reason, in our opinion, that endocavitary pacing is the method of choice even in young patients.

3. Pacing failure

In bipolar or unipolar stimulation the threshold is measured after disconnecting the pacemaker. If the threshold is normal and constant during tests designed to detect pacing failure, then the pacemaker box itself is suspect of having caused the breakdown. The electric parameters (amplitude, period times, duration of activation) may be measured using a sterile wire which is relayed to an oscilloscope. The replacement of a faulty or expired pacemaker is curative but many faults may coexist in the same patient.

If the threshold is raised on a bipolar catheter, a unipolar measurement may be carried out on each of the electrodes. This may permit satisfactory permanent pacing by **unipolar stimulation** if the threshold of one of the two electrodes is normal.

If the threshold is raised on both electrodes, the pacing catheter or the epicardio-myocardial electrodes must be replaced. Occasionally, the maximum amplitude of stimulation of the measuring pacemaker is inadequate using unipolar technique on one of the two electrodes of a bipolar catheter. This is the result of a break in the wire. A unipolar system may be connected on the other electrode. If the threshold is raised in milli-amperes on both wires using a unipolar technique, one is usually dealing with a short circuit between the two wires. A unipolar function is sometimes possible.

As a rule, a safety margin of at least 1·5 volts is observed between the threshold of the patient and the amplitude of the pacemaker.

When a unipolar electrode has a raised threshold and a radiological position which is too near the apex, perforation of the myocardium must be considered. A gentle withdrawal of the catheter under continuous external control may give normal threshold values. In other cases, the catheter has to be changed.

The fault may in some cases be due to a breakdown in the sensing circuit of the pacemaker. The amplitude of potential detected by the electrodes needs to be measured. One solution for a bipolar system is to connect the pacemaker as for a monopolar stimulation after having checked that a greater potential is obtained that when using the bipolar system. If this same fault occurs in a unipolar system, the electrode has to be changed.

D) DISCHARGE FROM HOSPITAL

When the patient leaves hospital, he should be advised to avoid too vigorous exercise of the arms. Golfers, tennis players and people who like swimming should moderate their activity. A complete check up is carried out at hospital which includes assessment of the pacemakers function. The patient is also advised about hygiene and his general way of life. He is given a **card** indicating that he is a pacemaker patient.

E) REPLACING A PACEMAKER

There are three situations in which a pacemaker needs to be replaced:

Firstly, prophylactically, when the average life span of the device draws to an end, and the patient for one reason or another cannot be closely followed up. Secondly, should there be electronic or electrocardiographic signs of running down or should the device break down for a reason unrelated to running down, replacement is indicated.

Replacing a pacemaker is a simpler procedure than the initial implantation. The pacemaker box is exposed and the connecting wire visualised. This is often a long, delicate and meticulous task as the wires are covered by a block of **fibrous tissue** which has to be dissected away little by little. The least damage to the protective envelope of the wire by scalpel or sissors will lead to a leak of current which will only become apparent long after. After the dissection, the **threshold of stimulation** is checked and then the new pacemaker is connected up. The disconnection of the original pacemaker should be carried out with caution as some patients, their illness being more evolved, do not exhibit spontaneous cardiac activity. In other words, **disconnection of the pacemaker will lead to a ventricular pause.** In some of these cases, a lazy idio-ventricular rhythm may be provoked by an intermittent contact between the pacing wire and one of the terminals of the pacemaker. A very slow rhythm of stimulation will be obtained which may lead to the reapparition of a ventricular rhythm. In other cases, this is not possible and for this reason, many operators prefer to change the pacemaker under cover of temporary pacing.

TYPICAL CHRONIC THRESHOLDS

Voltage	$1\cdot2 \pm 0\cdot3$ V
Current	$2\cdot1 \pm 0\cdot5$ mA

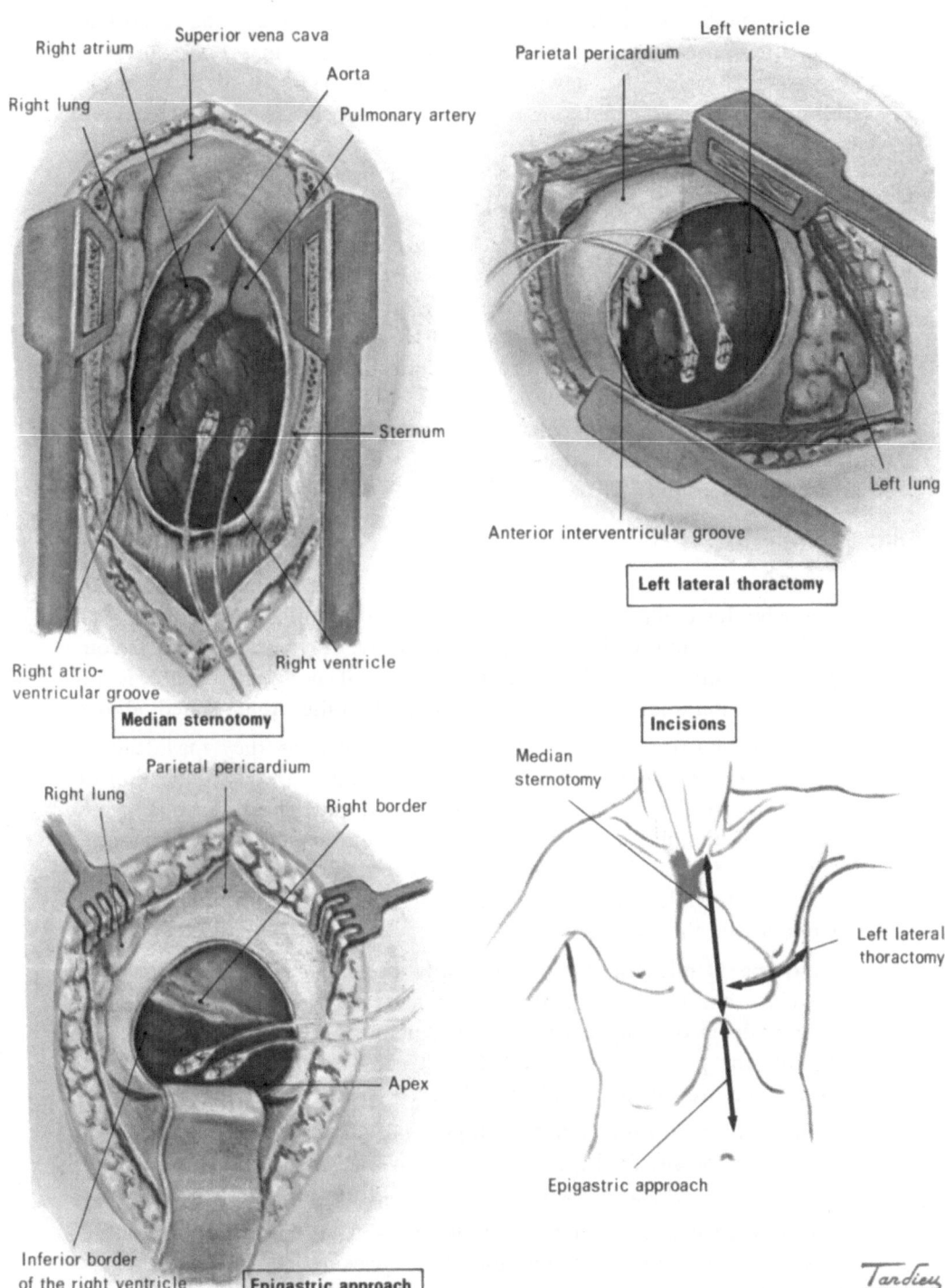

Right atrium
Superior vena cava
Aorta
Right lung
Pulmonary artery
Sternum
Right atrio-ventricular groove
Right ventricle

Median sternotomy

Parietal pericardium
Left ventricle
Anterior interventricular groove
Left lung

Left lateral thoractomy

Parietal pericardium
Right lung
Right border
Apex
Inferior border of the right ventricle

Epigastric approach

Incisions

Median sternotomy
Left lateral thoractomy
Epigastric approach

Tardieu

After implantation of a pacemaker, the patient may lead a normal active life for his age. The improvement is sometimes only observed after several weeks. Knowing that he is carrying a delicate intracorporal device responsible for regulating his cardiac rhythm, the patient will ask his doctor if there are any extrinsic situations which might upset its function, though he will no doubt be aware through the press or his friends of some of the risks.

Demand pacemakers contain a sensing circuit which is susceptible to electrical signals of the order of a thousandth of a volt. One might think that **external electromagnetic fields** might disrupt its function but this problem has been partially resolved by the manufacturers who have improved on the original electronic circuits by inserting selective filters and enclosing the electronic circuit in a protective metal envelope. Nevertheless, these improvements do not confer total security, and although most activities are permissable for the pacemaker patient, there are some environments, rarely encountered, which are hostile.

1. Every day situations that do not affect pacemakers

An active life is not contra-indicated for pacemaker patients, but those who have an A-V block will be more limited by shortness of breath on exertion which disappears at rest. They should be encouraged to accept a slightly diminished level of activity. There is no reason for limitation of a normal sexual life other than stated above.

Violent sporting activities are contra-indicated as they may lead to physical contact which may damage the electrodes or the connection of the pacing wire and pacemaker. More moderate sports such as golf, tennis or swimming are not formally contra-indicated nor encouraged. Walking is a good form of exercise. There is no limitation due to **altitude** and walks in the mountains are permitted. **Thunder storms** do not affect the pacemakers.

Driving is allowed, but should only be undertaken after the first pacemaker check up. The safety belt may be unconfortable for pacemaker patients on long journeys or frequent stops. It is recommended that only the part of the safety belt that goes around the waist is worn (The police are aware of this problem).

Different **motorised vehicles** should not affect pacemaker function but the patient should be advised to keep away from the high voltage electric circuits of cars, lawn mowers or motorcycles.

It has been shown that metal detectors as used by airport authorities to counter hijacking do not affect pacemakers and there is no other-contra-indication to air travel.

IMPLANTATION OF PERMANENT ENDOCAVITARY PACEMAKER
(Right cephalic venous approach through delto-pectoral skin incision)

1- Television monitor for radiological screening **2-** X-Ray machine
3- Continuous ECG monitoring with alarm system **4-** External pacemaker for measuring threshold
5- Sterile box of permanent pacemaker

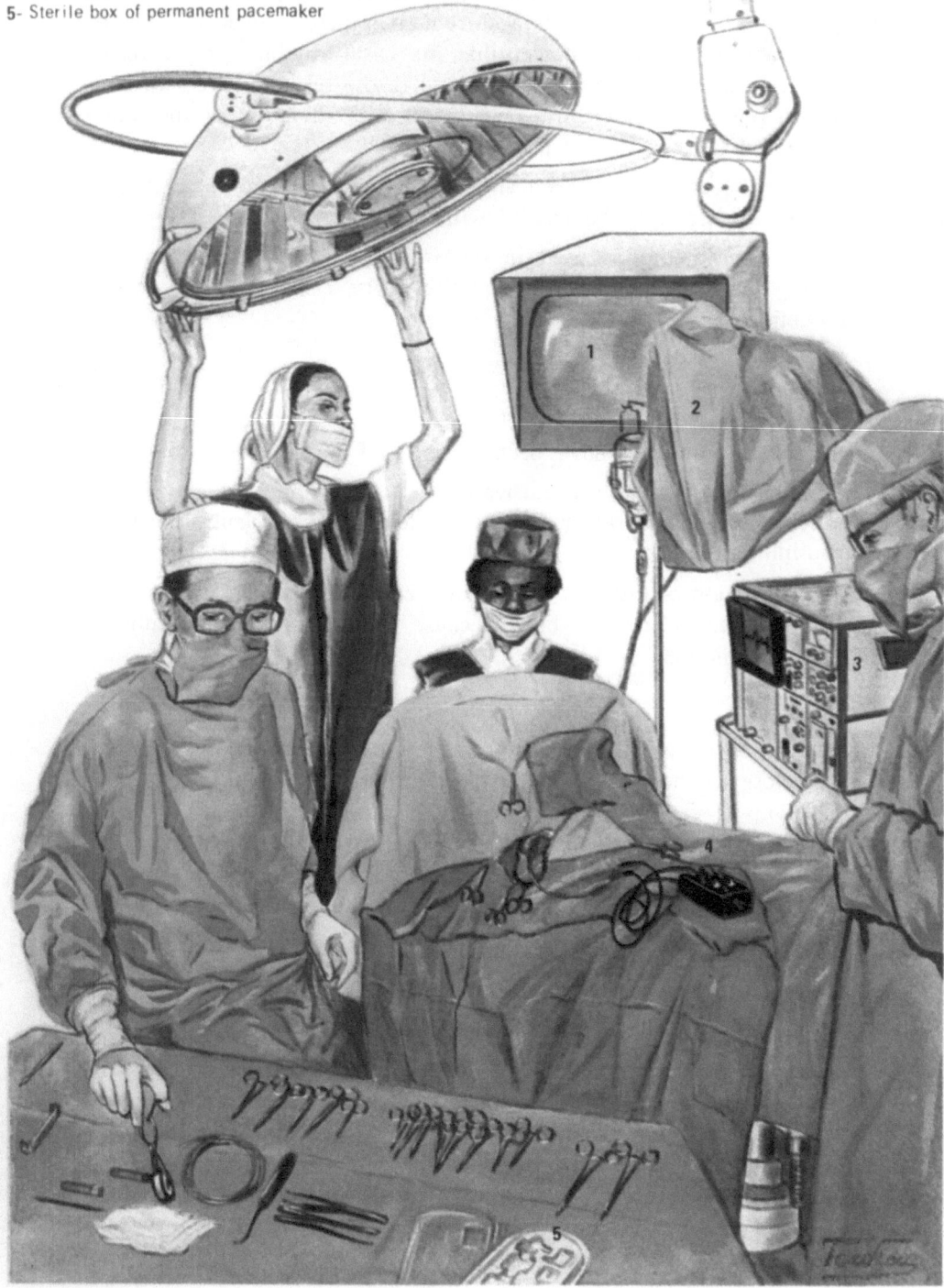

Electric household appliances were initially a cause of pacemaker inhibition. Only a small leakage of current from the devices earthed by the patient holding it, was sufficient to inhibit the pacemaker. Nowadays, if the pacemaker detects a current, it is programmed to function at a fixed rate, faster or slower than its basal rhythm. As a result, there is no danger from handling electric razors or hair dryers or even television sets. As for electric machinery, it is advised that the **motor is not placed** too near to the pacemaker.

There do not appear to be any contra-indications to drug therapy and other diseases may be treated without risk.

Local anaesthetics as used in minor surgery or dentistry are safe **providing** the pacing is of good quality. The same goes for general anaesthetics.

2. **Situations that may affect pacemakers**

a) *Endogenous*

Muscular potentials have been a cause of pacemaker dysfunction. This abnormality has been exclusively observed in **unipolar** pacing mode, contraction of the pectoralis major may be detected by the neutral electrode and so inhibit the pacemaker.

The detection of **P-waves** has in some cases of bipolar catheters with widely separated electrodes been a cause of intermittent inhibition of pacemaker function.

b) *Exogenous*

Micro-waves ovens: These new gadgets use a system of very short waves, close to that of radar, for cooking food. The electromagnetic field set up is very powerful and though when new, these appliances are equiped with a safety system to prevent leaks of the high frequency field, the use of an old oven not in perfect condition may upset pacemaker function. In the same way, **strong industrial electromagnetic fields** of high frequency are dangerous. Television or radio-transmitters may be dangerous if one passes close to the antennae. The risk is greater for radar stations. Police radar on the other hand is harmless.

In medico-surgical fields, the use of diathermy in surgery and electric scalpels or **transurethral resectors** may affect demand pacemakers. Precautions are necessary. A neutral electrode must be placed under the patient's buttocks and the trajectory of the wire connected to the diathermy should be at right angles to the pacemaker electrodes. Electrocardiographic monitoring is essential during the operation. Modern ECG machines have a floating input amplifier which is unaffected by the strong fields produced by the electric scalpel.

Defibrillation is possible due to the fact that pacemakers have a system which limits the risks of damage. To be quite sure, one of the defibrillator paddles should be placed on the back of the patient and the other on the chest. The risk of pacemaker dysfunction under these conditions is much greater with **extracorporal pacemakers** connected to a temporary pacing catheter. Telemetric monitoring devices or even electric razors may alter their function. In any case, any medical or surgical treatment of pacemaker patients should be carried out in the hospital where the pacemaker was implanted where a medical team is on call all around the clock.

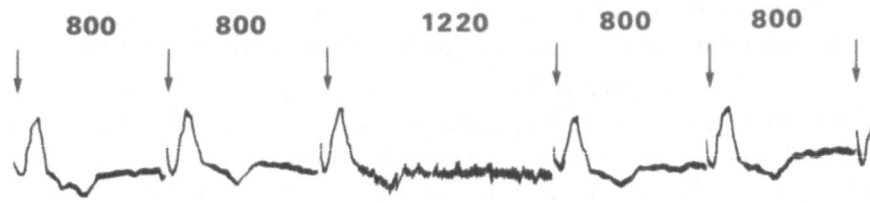

Muscular potential inhibition

FOLLOW-UP OF PACEMAKER PATIENTS

The doctor must be particularly vigilant in the first months after implantation. A careful note will be made on the way the patient has reacted to the pacemaker, both physically and psychologically. The doctor's knowledge and judgement will keep the patient from major complications, futile risks and unjustified hospitalisation.

A) CLINICAL FOLLOW-UP

1. General health

Reactions to the implantation vary from patient to patient and are often related to the circumstances under which it was carried out.

—The first category is that of the patient operated on as an emergency for repeated syncopal episodes, the serious nature of which he has realised and the reccurrence of which he feared. A few weeks after his operation he realises that the syncopes will not reccur and he is extremely grateful.

—The second category is that of the patient who presented with an history of tiredness, falls, and in some cases loss of consciousness over a number of months or years before implantation of a pacemaker. Again, a spectacular improvement may be observed although it may take one or two months.

—The third category is that of patient operated on prophylactically for paroxysmal A-V blocks presenting few symptoms. The pacemaker will be rarely in use and little or no improvement will be apparent.

—It is rare that a patient is worse off after implantation of a pacemaker. However, when a patient with a sino-atrial block is paced from the ventricle a **retrograde 1/1 depolarisation** of the atrium may have unfavourable haemodynamic effects usually manifest as a dyspnoea of effort. Finally, some patients have an uncomfortable sensation when a demand pacemaker starts pacing, though functioning quite normally (this is especially so with epicardial electrodes).

2. Heart failure

This is a frequent problem in pacemaker patients for several reasons. There is a dissociation between the atrial and ventricular contraction in a patient in A-V block who is permanently paced, which deprives the ventricles of the benefit of atrial contraction. In certain cases, this represents 20 % to 40 % of the cardiac output. Also the ventricular contraction of a paced beat is less physiological and may give rise to or aggravate mitral incompetence, previously asymptomatic. This haemo-

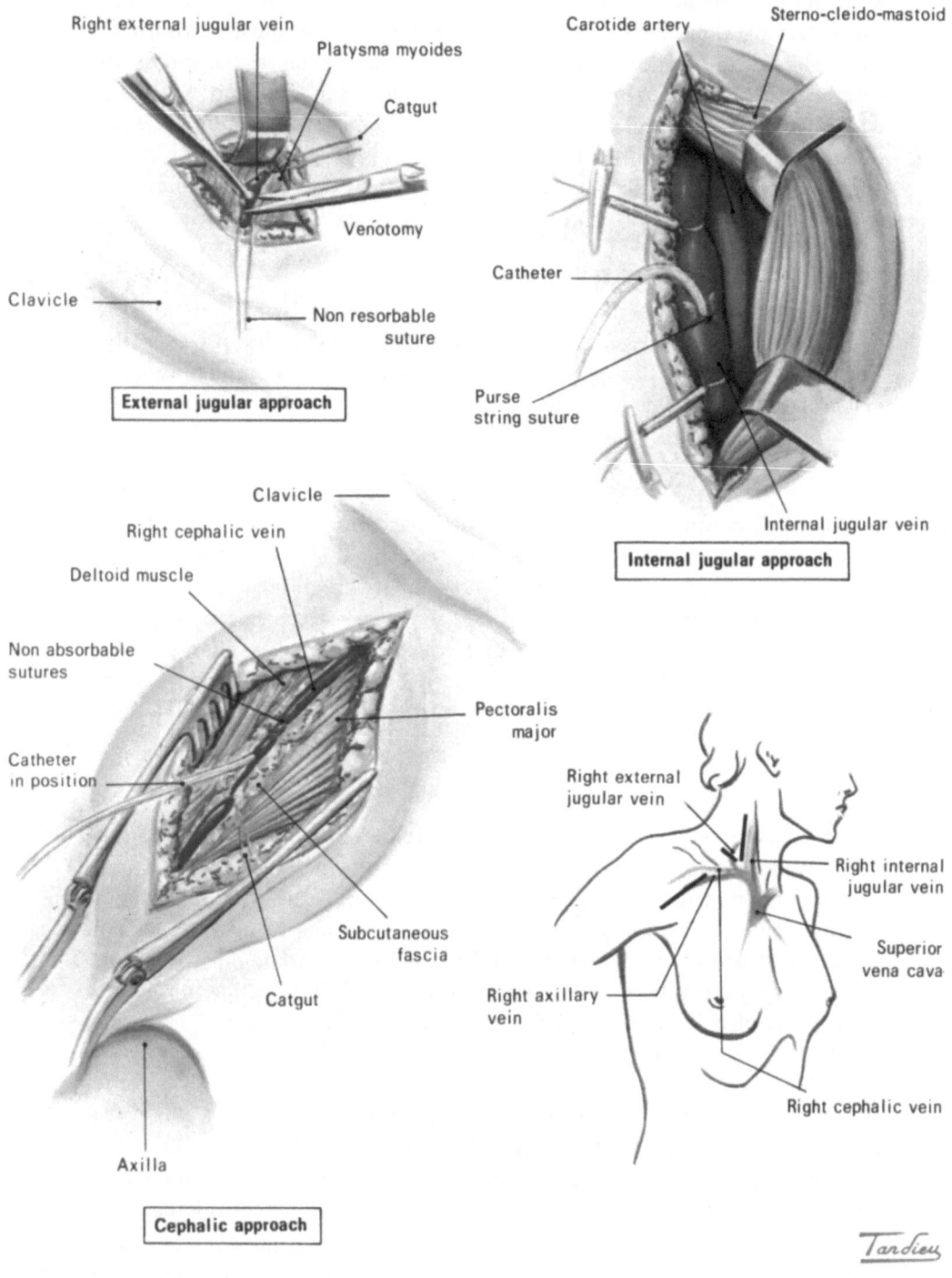

External jugular approach

Right external jugular vein
Platysma myoides
Catgut
Venotomy
Clavicle
Non resorbable suture

Internal jugular approach

Carotide artery
Sterno-cleido-mastoid
Catheter
Purse string suture
Internal jugular vein

Cephalic approach

Clavicle
Right cephalic vein
Deltoid muscle
Non absorbable sutures
Catheter in position
Pectoralis major
Subcutaneous fascia
Catgut
Axilla

Right external jugular vein
Right internal jugular vein
Superior vena cava
Right axillary vein
Right cephalic vein

Tardieu

55

dynamic alteration is usually well compensated during hospitalisation when the patient is at rest. However in the weeks following discharge either left or right heart failure may develop. This must be born in mind should the patient consult with symptoms such as shortness of breath, tiredness, or **peripheral oedema.** A low salt diet and treatment with digoxin and diuretics and potassium supplements should be instituted. The patient should be followed up closely until the problem is under control. In some patients, the pacemaker rate may be increased to 80 or 90/min and this may lead to a temporary improvement.

3. Respiratory insufficiency

Shortness of breath may be a presenting symptom which if not due to heart failure, may be related to a restriction of respiratory capacity. The cause may be a **post-pericardiotomy syndrome** after implantation of epicardial electrodes or the removal of infected epicardial electrodes.

4. Coronary insufficiency

Signs of coronary artery disease may be present before A-V block and remain after implantation of the pacemaker. Aggravation may occur due to the reduction in cardiac output in the absence of a normal A.-V sequence. In these patients, the frequency of the pacemaker may be reduced to between 60-65/min and current anti-anginal therapy with beta blockers may be prescribed. These drugs may be prescribed at larger doses than those normally used as the pacemaker avoids their main side effect, that of bradycardia.

5. Skin reactions

It is essential to check on the **state of the skin** in the first months after implantation. Depending on the patient, the pacemaker is implanted either in the subcutaneous tissue, or behind the pectoralis major but its weight or anatomical position sometimes leads to **migration** from the original site of implantation. This is extremely common in patients with heavy pacemakers (mercury batteries) and it is quite normal to find the device in a lower site after a few weeks.

6. Pain

Pain may be felt at the site of the pacemaker box or at the point of entry of the pacing catheter into the external jugular vein. The skin is often red and oedematous. This situation may be an inflammatory reaction to a foreign body but infection must always be considered.

When these signs last for more than a week and the skin becomes red, shiney and extremely tender, infection of the pacemaker is the most likely diagnosis and a short period of hospitalisation is indicated.

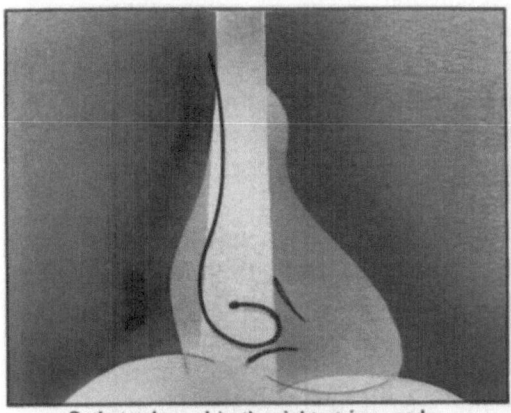

Catheter looped in the right atrium ready
to cross the tricuspid valve.

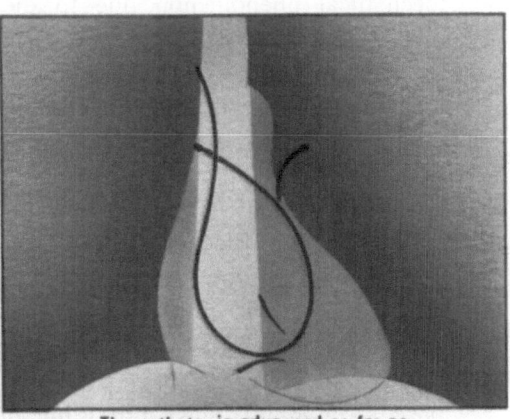

The catheter is advanced as far as
the pulmonary artery.

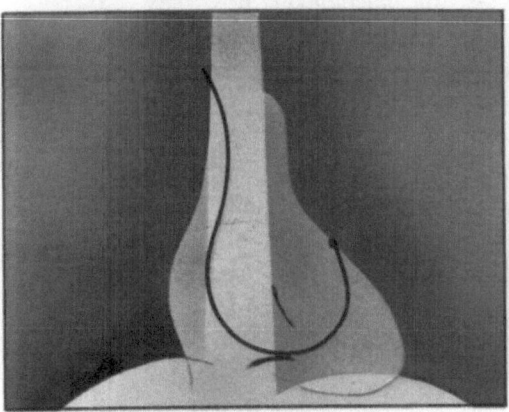

Withdrawal of the catheter along
the wall of the infundibulum.

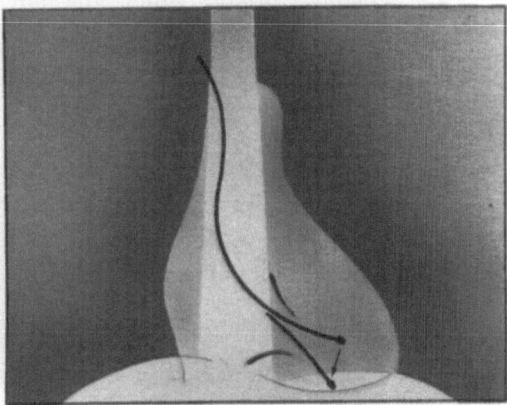

The catheter falls to the floor
of the right ventricle.

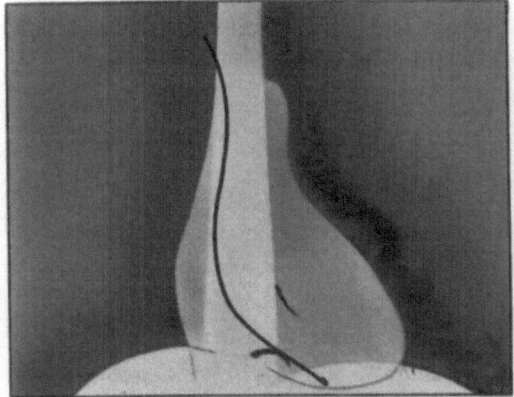

The catheter is then advanced to
the paratricuspid area.

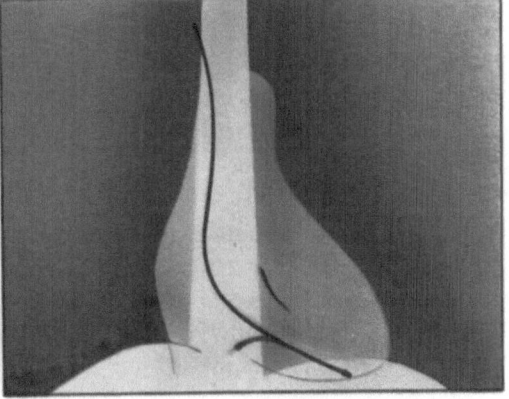

The catheter is then advanced to the apex

Tardieu

Another type of pain may be experienced which is secondary to a mechanical phenomenon due to the rectangular shape of some pacemakers. A localised red tender area with a reduction in subcutaneous tissue at the **angles** of the pacemaker box will be apparent. These signs may develop slowly after several months or even a year after implantation. In other patients, a thinning of the skin and subcutaneous tissue may develop much more rapidly at the point where the pacemaker juts out. The patient must be sent to a specialised centre without delay as the pacemaker "pocket" is **still sterile** and the operation needed will only involve burying the pacemaker a little more deeply. If things are left to take their course the pacemaker will become more and more superficial until after a certain interval the skin breaks down with a serous exudate. In some cases, it is still possible to re-implant the pacemaker at this stage providing that the area is not infected. More often, signs of infection are present and an erythematous zone surrounds the wound through which the angle of the pacemaker box may be observed surrounded by a yellowish fluid. In this case, re-implantation of the whole pacemaker system must be carried out on the opposite side.

7. **Hematomas**

These usually occur in the early post-operative period and may present in two different ways: The first picture is that of a diffuse superficial hemorrhage involving a large skin area from the zone of implantation and extending along the arm down the chest and over part of the abdomen. These hematomas are quite spectacular but are not serious and usually disappear spontaneously in a couple of weeks.

The second presentation is that of a localised hematoma due to a haemorrhage around the pacemaker case. It may develop after early reinstitution of anti-coagulant therapy or in patients with a clotting defect. This type of hematoma is **more serious** and requires daily or twice daily checks and necessitates a period of hospitalisation. Aspiration of the hematoma must only be carried out under surgical conditions otherwise infection may be introduced.

8. **Thromboses**

Venous thrombosis of the arm on the side of the endocavitary catheter is a rare complication, more spectacular than painful, which presents with severe oedema. Anti-coagulants may be prescribed especially if a thrombo-embolic incident occurs but in the main the condition resolves spontaneously without long term sequelae in a few weeks.

9. **Muscular stimulations**

There are several forms:

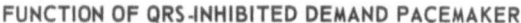

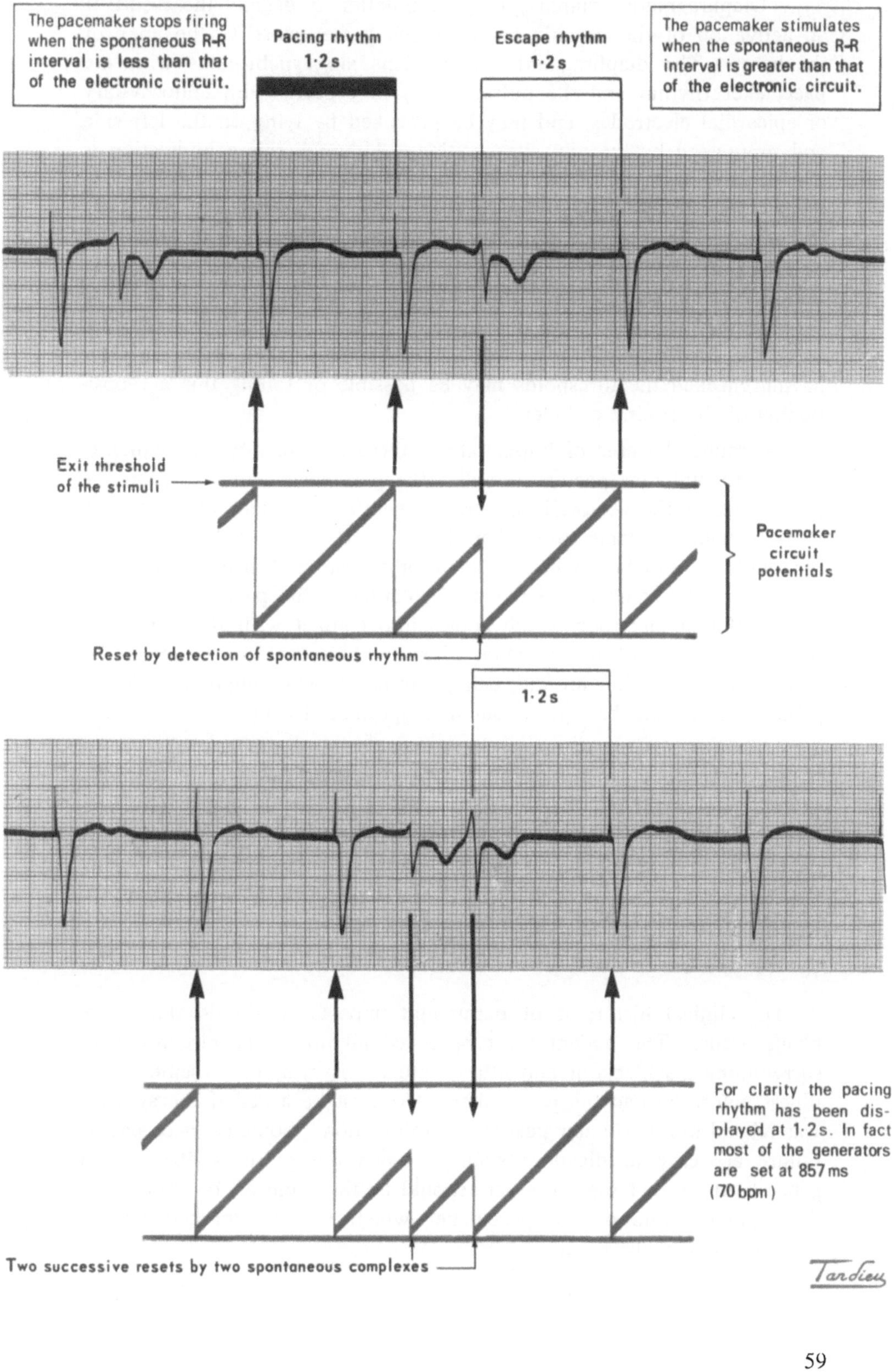

The pacemaker stops firing when the spontaneous R-R interval is less than that of the electronic circuit.

Pacing rhythm
1·2 s

Escape rhythm
1·2 s

The pacemaker stimulates when the spontaneous R-R interval is greater than that of the electronic circuit.

Exit threshold of the stimuli →

Pacemaker circuit potentials

Reset by detection of spontaneous rhythm

1·2 s

For clarity the pacing rhythm has been displayed at 1·2 s. In fact most of the generators are set at 857 ms (70 bpm)

Two successive resets by two spontaneous complexes

Tardieu

59

—Diaphragmatic: diaphragmatic stimulation is usually the result of an activation of the phrenic nerve, which passes close to the apex of the heart. The diaphragmatic contractions are **synchronous with the pacemaker** rhythm and the pulse. They may occur with endocavitary or epicardial electrodes, and may be provoked by lying on the left side and suppressed by the opposite position. Although this complication is not dangerous it may lead to insomnia. They are easily reproduced during the clinical examination by putting a magnet against the pacemaker if the heart rate inhibits the pacemaker. There are several ways of solving this problem. The amplitude of stimulation may be reduced (programmable pacemakers) providing a sufficient margin of security between the threshold value and the amplitude of stimulation is allowed. A simple inversion of the polarity of a bipolar pacing catheter after having checked the thresholds may be possible or failing this a repositioning of the pacing catheter.

—Around the area of implantation: these problems quite frequently occur with unipolar pacing should if the pacemaker box has been implanted under the pectoralis major. Generally, the signs occur after a week or two. In some cases, they develop early, around the pacemaker box with a unipolar catheter which otherwise had been functioning normally. The cause may be that of rotation of the pacemaker around the indifferent electrode which comes into contact with the muscle or the ramifications of the brachial plexus. This may be corrected by turning the pacemaker around, using a transcutaneous approach. These manoeuvres should be carried out in a specialised centre.

—Around the pacing wires, or the pacemaker of a bipolar system: if this occurs it is usually due to an **electrical leak** through the isolating plastic envelope of the pacing wire. This must be looked for with care the whole length of the electrode from its point of insertion into the pacemaker. In this type of pacing, muscular stimulation is a pathognomonic sign of leak. The ECG will show a clear variation in the amplitude of the spike.

10. Blackouts and syncopes

The clinical history is of paramount importance should these problems occur. The patient must be asked all about the circumstances **surrounding** his blackout and also whether this symptom resembled his illness **before** he had the pacemaker. He must be asked if the syncope was related to a particular position or to exertion. Some cases of pacing failure are easy to diagnose such as when the pulse is 40/min. A general rule is that the pulse rate should be the same as, or faster than the regulated rate of the pacemaker which will be marked on the patient's pacemaker card.

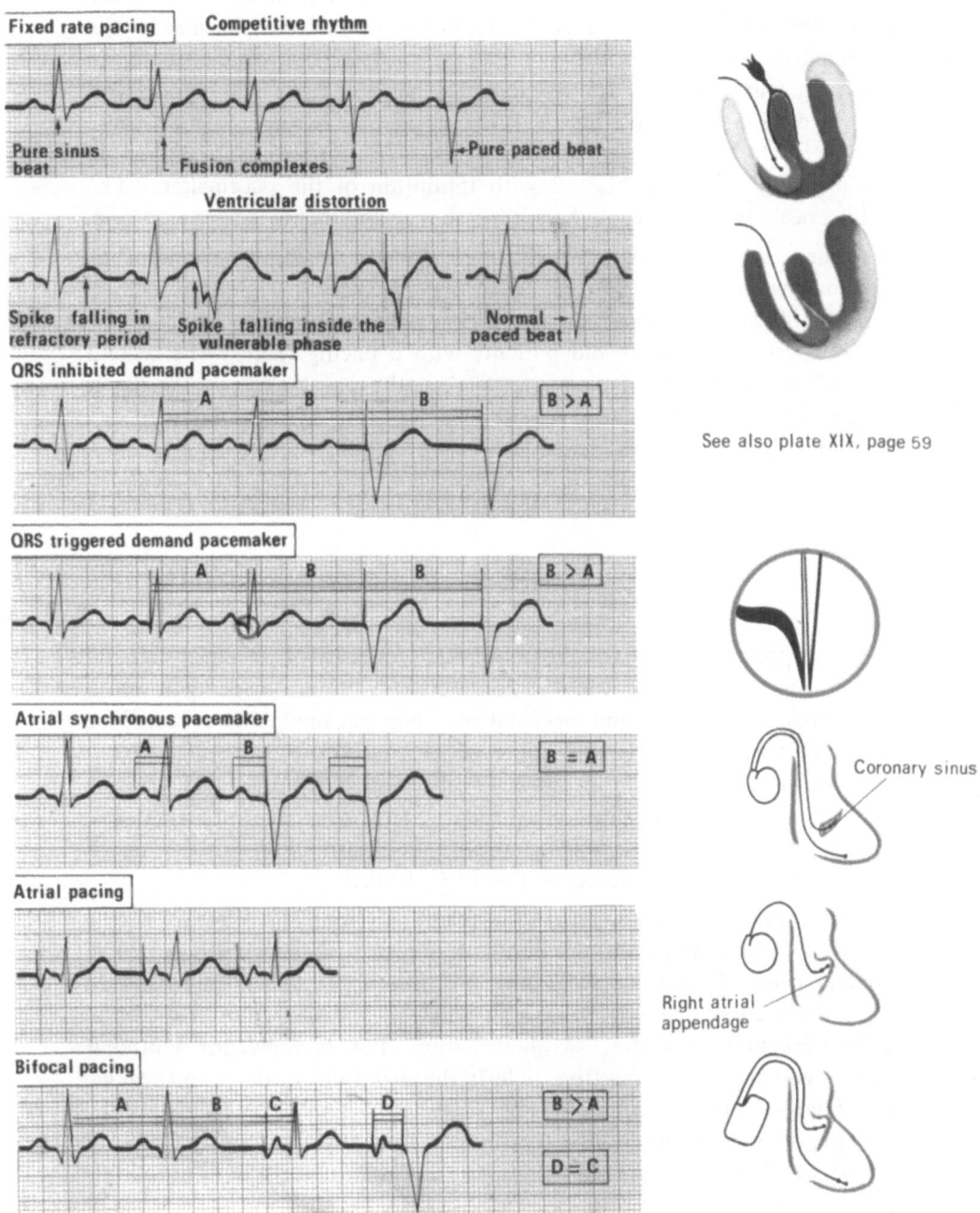

Fixed rate pacing — **Competitive rhythm**

Pure sinus beat — Fusion complexes — Pure paced beat

Ventricular distortion

Spike falling in refractory period — Spike falling inside the vulnerable phase — Normal paced beat

QRS inhibited demand pacemaker

A — B — B — B > A

QRS triggered demand pacemaker

A — B — B — B > A

Atrial synchronous pacemaker

A — B — B = A

Atrial pacing

Bifocal pacing

A — B — C — D — B > A — D = C

See also plate XIX, page 59

Coronary sinus

Right atrial appendage

Tardieu

Most mercury powered pacemakers have a life of 27 to 40 months and lithium batteries have a life span of about 5 years. A slowing of the rhythm (from 70 to 60/min) is the criterion most often used. When the rhythm is regular at the regulated rate of the pacemaker, the pacemaker may be checked by putting a transistor radio, tuned between two long wave stations, against the pacemaker. Each stimulation will be heard as a "bip-bip" on the loud speaker. If the patient's pulse rate is faster than the rate of the pacemaker, normal A-V conduction has probably been restablished with inhibition of the pacemaker. The radio check will be negative, except in certain makes of pacemakers.

When the pacemaker is inhibited by the patient's spontaneous rhythm, two methods exist to check its efficacity. The first method consists of cardiac sinus massage with vagal stimulation. This is not without risk especially in old patients with a pacing fault. The second method is the placing of a **magnet** against the pacemaker so causing it to stimulate at a fixed rate. It will then interfere with the spontaneous rhythm.

B) THE ECG IN PACEMAKER PATIENTS

1. Normal ECG (Plate XX, p 61)

a) *Permanent and continuous ventricular pacing*

This type of recording is the one most frequently observed in patients without normal atrio-ventricular conduction who are dependent on a fixed rhythm or a demand pacemaker. The pacemaker is revealed as a stimulation artefact called a **spike** which precedes the paced complex. In bipolar stimulation, the spike is of small amplitude and so, the ventricular morphology may be studied. However, in unipolar stimulation, its amplitude is great, masking the morphology of the paced ventricular complex in some of the ECG leads.

The spike is a fine deflection resulting from the electric dipole created by the impulse of stimulation at the tips of the electrodes. The general rules of electrocardiography are thus applicable. There should be a correlation between the dipole angle calculated from the frontal ECG derivations and the P-A chest X-ray. For example, for a bipolar pacing catheter whose negative pole is the distal electrode, a spike angle of about — 110° (± 15°) will be recorded. This axis may vary by 15° to 30° with respiration. In this case, projection along the axis of LLIII which is almost perpendicular will lead to variations in its amplitude (sometimes to its inversion).

The morphology of the paced QRS complex is always wide as it corresponds in part to a ventricular extrasystole arising from the point of stimulation. With epicardial electrodes placed in the left ventricular

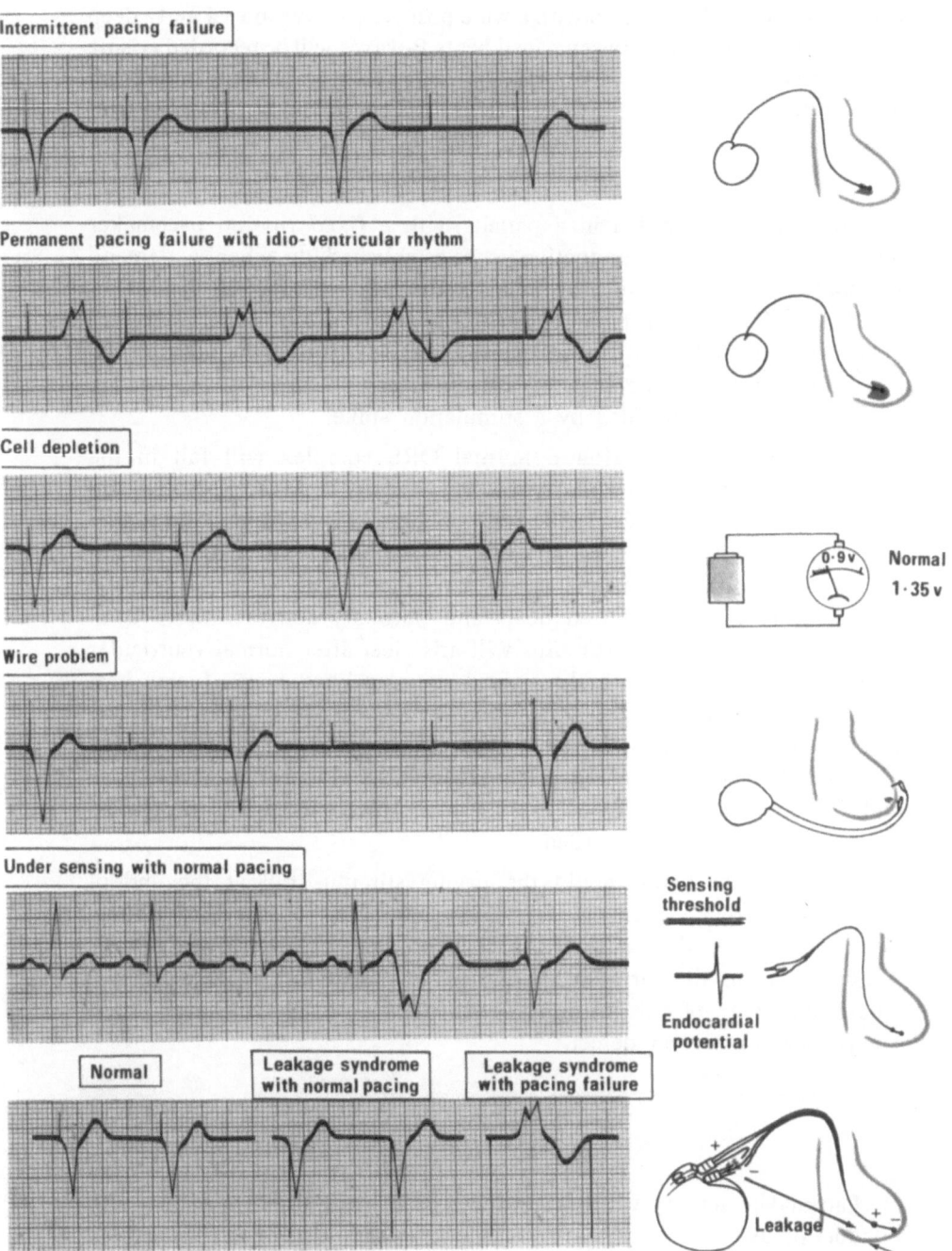

Intermittent pacing failure

Permanent pacing failure with idio-ventricular rhythm

Cell depletion

Normal
1·35 v

Wire problem

Under sensing with normal pacing

Sensing threshold

Endocardial potential

Normal | Leakage syndrome with normal pacing | Leakage syndrome with pacing failure

Leakage

Tardieu

wall the ECG tracing will be that of **delayed right** sided activation, and for an endocavitary catheter, placed at the apex of the right ventricle, a **delayed left** sided activation with a wide positive R-wave in LLI and a deep QS in LLII and LLIII. Between paced beats P-waves will be recorded arising at their own rhythm. They will not be followed by a ventricular response and will appear to separate progressively from the paced rhythm.

b) *Interference rhythm*

This may be recorded in a patient with a fixed rhythm pacemaker when atrio-ventricular conduction is re-established or when a demand pacemaker is made to function at a fixed rhythm by the application of a magnet. Two major types of recording may be observed:

—Normal P-QRS sequences when the activation uses the normal A-V conduction system to depolarise the ventricles.

—Paced beats preceded by a stimulation spike.

Some spikes arising after a normal QRS complex will fall in the refractory period and so will not be followed by a paced complex and reciprocally some P-waves will not command a ventricular response. The rhythm of the pacemaker and that of the sinus node being different, during a period of interference rhythm, there will be a progressive separation between the paced beats and normally activated QRS complexes. Rarely the paced stimulus will arise just after normal ventricular depolarisation has started and a hybrid complex known as a **fusion beat** will result. Its morphology will resemble the start of a normal depolarisation and then, after the spike, the rest of the complex will be that of a paced beat. According to the time interval between the P-wave and the spike, a whole range of fusion complexes from the normal to a paced beat, may be recorded.

On the other hand should the pacing stimulus fall at the end of a normally activated ventricular depolarisation or conversely a normal activation fall at the end of a paced complex, the ventricle may be re-excited during the period of repolarisation (relative refractory period). The morphology of the resulting complex will be altered by an intraventricular conduction defect.

c) *The ECG of a demand pacemaker patient*

● QRS inhibited

Pacemaker activity will not be observed in patients with normal A-V conduction as long as the heart rate is greater than that of the pacemaker. This leads to difficulty in checking the integrity of the pacing system. The problem may be solved by the use of a **magnet** placed against the pacemaker which activates a magnetic switch causing the pacemaker to

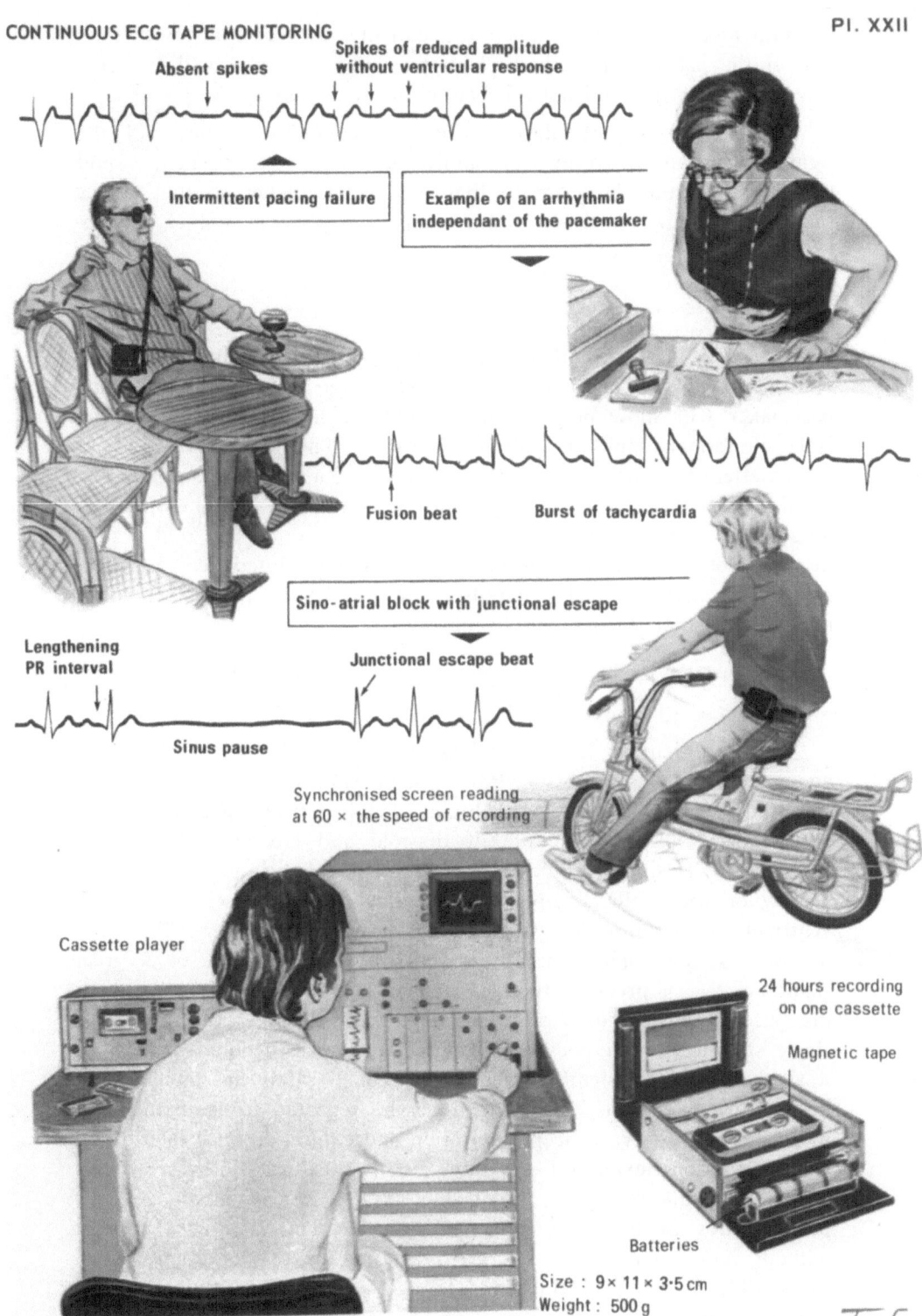

Absent spikes

Spikes of reduced amplitude without ventricular response

Intermittent pacing failure

Example of an arrhythmia independant of the pacemaker

Fusion beat   Burst of tachycardia

Sino-atrial block with junctional escape

Lengthening PR interval

Junctional escape beat

Sinus pause

Synchronised screen reading at 60 × the speed of recording

Cassette player

24 hours recording on one cassette

Magnetic tape

Batteries

Size : 9 × 11 × 3·5 cm
Weight : 500 g

Tardieu

65

function at a fixed rate. When the patient's own rate is lower than that of the pacemaker, spikes which pace the ventricles will be seen. The ventricular rate will not fall below that regulated by the pacemaker.

In some cases, particularly those with conduction defects of the right branch and antero-superior ramifications of the left branch, should the sinusal rhythm be close to that of the pacemaker so that spikes fall in the normally activated QRS complex, a phenomenon of **pseudo-fusion** will be observed.

- QRS triggered

The recording of a patient with a QRS triggered demand pacemaker with normal A-V conduction at a rhythm greater than that of the pacemaker will show normal QRS complexes in which a stimulation spike of normal amplitude will be observed. This spike arrives about 10 ms **after** the start of the QRS complex and a simultaneous ECG of the three standard leads is necessary to check that the stimulation really does occur after the beginning of normal depolarisation and that it falls in the absolute refractory period. As in QRS inhibited demand pacemakers, when the normal rate falls below that of the pacemaker continuous ventricular pacing will be observed.

2. **ECG abnormalities in pacemaker patients** (Plate XXI, p 63)

   a) *Ventricular pacing faults*

The most frequent fault is of loss of contact between the electrodes and myocardium. The ECG shows pacing spikes of normal axis and amplitude compared to those obtained with normal pacing. However, some fall in the middle of diastole and are not followed by a QRS complex. The underlying rhythm may be sinusal with either narrow or wide QRS complexes depending on the presence of intraventricular conduction defects, or it may be idio-ventricular. The finding of a **solitary** spike without a ventricular response is of a great significance. In practice, there is a large margin of security between the pacemaker amplitude and the ventricular diastolic threshold. A **single stimulus** which does not lead to ventricular depolarisation even if all the others do, signifies that the margin of safety has momentarily been reduced to zero. The ECG must be repeated using methods of increasing sensitivity, in deep inspiration and expiration with lateral and antero-posterior flexions of the thorax, hyperflexions of the neck and during manipulation of the pacemaker (under ECG control) and the pacing wires in their subcutaneous tunnel. The finding of spikes without ventricular response is an indication for re-operation as soon as possible as the problem tends to **aggravate** until complete pacing failure occurs.

When the fault is due to a higher threshold than the stimulating power of the pacemaker, an impulse arriving at the end of the T-wave may still obtain a ventricular response (super-normal phase). These faults necessitate re-operation to reposition the electrodes. In some cases, the fault is sometimes intermittent rather than constant and may pose diagnostic problems. This situation justifies long derivation recording or Holter monitoring.

b) *Fault of the sensing circuit*

This problem only concerns demand pacemakers when the sensing circuit **fails to pick up spontaneous QRS complexes.** In its usual form the ECG shows stimulation spikes occuring after the spontaneous QRS complexes which have not been detected. This fault may be intermittent, only being recorded in parts of the ECG. In a more serious form, a fault in the sensing circuit may give rise to an interference rhythm. This fault may be associated with a fault in the pacing circuit where some spikes do not obtain ventricular response. When the fault occurs shortly after the positioning of an endocavitary catheter, it is often a precursory sign of a **pacing defect.** If the fault occurs near the end of the life of the pacemaker, it is a late sign of battery depletion.

c) *Faults due to rupture of the pacing wires*

This problem is rare with endocavitary catheters. Two types may be observed:

—Rupture of the pacing wire in its isolating covering. This is characterised by a complete absence of spikes or the presence of **minuscule spikes.** Usually, there is no ventricular response. When the spikes are visible they occur at the usual frequency.

—Rupture of the isolating covering without a break in the pacing wire. In this instance, the ECG is modified by the leakage of electric current which produces a **new electric** dipole with the electrode of opposite polarity. A modification of the amplitude and axis of the spike in the bipolar derivations is usually observed (the leak syndrome). This leak of current may be too small to interfere with normal ventricular pacing but nevertheless re-operation is necessary because the cause of rupture of the isolating covering may sever the pacing wire itself so causing a permanent pacing failure.

d) *Pacemaker failures*

These vary according to the causative mechanism, battery or electronic circuit. A detailed **oscilloscopic** analysis of the stimulation impulse as recorded on the standard ECG derivation is essential to determine whether a diminution of amplitude or an abnormality of the duration of the stimulatory period·exists. In some cases, the **stimulation**

period may be faster than normal. The most advanced forms, when the pacemaker rhythm rises to 200 or 250/min with its consequent danger should the amplitude of stimulation be sufficient to pace the ventricle, are practically never seen nowadays. In other cases, the pacemaker rhythm may be too slow and its rate may vary erratically.

C) RADIOLOGICAL INVESTIGATIONS

Radioscopic examination, if possible with screening, is advised as a routine, above all in the first months after implantation. Some pacing failures are easily diagnosed by a displacement of the pacing catheter which may be positioned in the pulmonary infundibulum, the right atrium or the inferior or superior vena cava with a loop of pacing wire around the pacing box.

Should the position of the pacing catheter be satisfactory, the study of its movements throughout the cardiac contraction may be informative. To and fro movements in the axis of the catheter or pendular movements of several centimeters in the ventricular cavity are significant. These different movements should be checked for in **deep inspiration and expiration.** Though often compatible with a satisfactory quality of pacing the abnormalities should be communicated to the centre where the pacemaker was implanted.

Radiography permits a more detailed examination of the pacing wires. This is not justified as a routine examination but is of great use when there is a pacing defect. Two different radiographic incidences are needed with strong penetration (as for a barium swallow radiograph). The **exposure time must be short** as the electrodes move with the heart. This sort of X-ray is too "hard" to visualise the lung fields but allows inspection of the length of the pacing wire. Epicardial electrodes are more susceptible to rupture than endocavitary catheters, the part most at risk being an acute angle at the distal extremity of the electrode, an area where the spiral wire is stretched. An eventual solution might be a continuity on one wire by angulation of two adjacent parts. Any suspicious angulation on X-ray should be checked by screening with the patient lying down, and in flexion in deep inspiration and expiration. It is to be noted however that some ruptures of the pacing wire do **not show up** on X-ray like distal ruptures between the pacing wire and the electrode of some bipolar pacing catheters).

D) CHECK-UP IN SPECIALISED CENTRES

Specialised centres are equiped with electronic devices which permit a more precise testing of the electric properties of pacemakers. The

When the magnet is applied the pacing rate is increased

Normal   NI   NI   Fusion beat   NI

Sinus rhythm inhibiting the P.M.

Spikes falling in refractory period

Inverted P waves showing retrograde conduction

Digital comptometer to measure electrical parameters

Triple channel ECG

Oscilloscope for wave form contour analysis

Pacemaker spike recorded from the surface ECG on the oscilloscope

50 mv

0·5ms

Tardieu

69

electric parameters may even be changed without risk to the patient. Their main function is (1) to determine the beginning of depletion of the batteries using objective criteria so that their replacement may be carried out at an opportune moment, not too soon so that the energy source of the pacemaker is used to its maximum and not too late so that the patient does not run needless risks, (2) to analyse and decide on management of abnormalities of pacemaker function (Plate XXIII, p 69).

The stimulation impulse of the pacemaker is poorly conducted through the human body but it is of sufficient amplitude to be detected on the surface by electronic devices. This impulse is responsible for the spike artefact of the ECG. After amplification these impulses may be studied by exact electronic means.

a) **Periodemeter**

This is an electronic counter which measures with greater precision than an ordinary ECG the time interval between two successive impulses. The paper speed of an ECG is regulated by a mechanical motor which may be inconstant, especially in portable machines. The periodemeter is an electronic instrument which is capable of measuring to **1/10th of a millisecond.** The long term follow up of these measurement gives a good indication of the state of the pacemaker battery as in most cases the characteristic feature of its deterioration is a slowing up of the pacemaker with a prolongation of the interspike interval.

With mercury powered pacemakers it is not unusual to observe a phenomenon of **drift,** that is to say a variation of several milliseconds more or less, during the first months. This phenomenon stabilises or reduces itself after a few months. The usage of the batteries is distinguished easily by an abrupt change of the order of **50 to 100 ms.** Several days or weeks later this variation increases and becomes clinically detectable. The rhythm of the pacemaker changes from 70 to 60/min.

With lithium powered pacemakers the variation of the interval is very **slow and progressive** and allows the doctor to estimate the remaining life span. These batteries are a recent innovation and confirmation of their properties by clinical observation is required.

Some of these instruments are capable of measuring the duration of the stimulus based on a similar principle but of greater precision, as intervals of up to a hundredth of a millisecond (1/100 ms) are measured. In most pacemakers the duration of stimulus **increases** at the time that the batteries start to run down.

The pacemaker stimulus as observed in the usual ECG derivations is projected on a cathode-ray oscilloscope. The sweep speed of the horizontal hold is adjusted between 0·1 ms to 1 ms, in order that the stimulus may be easily seen. The amplitude of a small spike of a bipolar catheter would be in the order of 10 to 20 millivolts for each vertical division and in the order of a 100 to 200 mv (large spikes) for monopolar stimulation. In this way, the **morphology** of the stimulus, which should remain the same at each check up, may be studied. Its amplitude may vary according to the position of the electrodes in the thorax, and notably with respiration. For this reason, this parameter is somewhat inconstant, if only recorded on one ECG derivation. A more precise measurement of the amplitude may be made by the simultaneous recording of two or better three derivations, and by calculating the mean from these three values. The oscilloscope is able to measure the interval between two spikes by using a horizontal sweep of about 100 ms by division, but the measurement is less exact than that of the periodemeter.

c) **The magnet test**

This test **converts** demand pacemakers, which are inhibited by a faster spontaneous rhythm **to a fixed rhythm**. This, of course, is the first check of an inhibited pacemaker before going on to measure the electrical parameters or carry out oscilloscopic analysis. However, the effect of the magnet may differ according to the type of pacemaker used. In some models (Cordis) the frequency of the spike is identical to the spontaneous pacemaker rhythm. In other models (Medtronic) the magnet rhythm is between 30 and 40 ms, slower than the spontaneous rhythm, and again for other models, the rhythm of stimulation is increased. For example, a pacemaker (CPI) which functions normally at 70/min will increase to 100/min (590 ms interval). In other models (Elema vario-pacer) the magnet test gives rise to a fixed rhythm associated with an acceleration and a progressive diminution of the amplitude of stimulation in fifteen steps.

The threshold may thus be measured in a non-invasive way. The characteristics therefore vary from one mark of pacemaker to another, and for this reason details of the pacemaker should be known by the patient or even better marked on his pacemaker patient card, which should be kept on his person at all times.

d) **Programmable pacemakers**

In some cases of cardiac arrhythmias, such as ventricular tachycardia, or heart failure or coronary insufficiency, it is often useful to be able to adjust the frequency of stimulation of the pacemaker. Some kinds of pacemakers may now be programmed externally. An electronic circuit with an independant power source which gives rise to a series of electromagnetic impulses is contained in the pacemaker. These impulses are decoded by the pacemaker so allowing the parameters of stimulation to be changed. After reprogramming the pacemaker the result must be checked using a periodemeter or an oscilloscope to ensure that the pacemaker has correctly interpreted the manipulation. The new parameters must be entered on the pacemaker patient card.

The same method may be used to change the amplitude and in these cases, a programing which preserves a good margin of security between the patient's threshold and the maximum amplitude of the pacemaker will be used. By this means, a rough idea of the threshold value may be obtained which is useful should the patient present with blackouts or syncopal episodes.

e) **Voluntary inhibition of an implanted pacemaker**

In some patients presenting either with arrhythmias or chest pain suggestive of myocardial infarction, it may be useful to inhibit the pacemaker to record the underlying rhythm and study the morphology of the ventriculogram. This must only be done under continuous electrocardiographical monitoring. There are two possible methods: either using a radio-frequency transmitter which gives out a pulsatile electromagnetic field, or using a stimulation by a weak current applied across the surface of the thorax, between two precordial ECG electrodes. These electric or electromagnetic fields, when adjusted to a frequency slightly more rapid than that of the pacemaker, are capable of completely inhibiting it so as to show up the underlying spontaneous rhythm of the patient (providing one exists!).

f) **The pacemaker patient booklet**

All pacemaker patients should be in possession of a booklet on which the main details of the implantation should be recorded. The personal identification of the patient, the names of his doctor and cardiologist and of the hospital where he was operated on, should be clearly noted. The date of the first implantation, the date of the positioning of the electrodes, the make and model of pacemaker used, the number of pacemakers that have been used on the working electrode, the characteristics of the pacemaker function, that is to say the make, the number of the model, the manufacturer's number, and in addition its basic properties, such as fixed rhythm or demand, the result of the magnet test and the possibility of programing the pacemaker, should be clearly indicated. On the other pages, the dates of the checks-up, the name of the doctors, the number of months that the

1 The antenna detects the electrical activity of the pacemaker through the patient's clothes.

2 The sound signal, synchronous with the pacemaker's impulse, is transmitted by the microphone in the telephone receiver

3 Reception equipment. The inter-spike interval is calculated in milliseconds.
(an ECG recording is not shown with this particular set-up)

4 Patient's records.

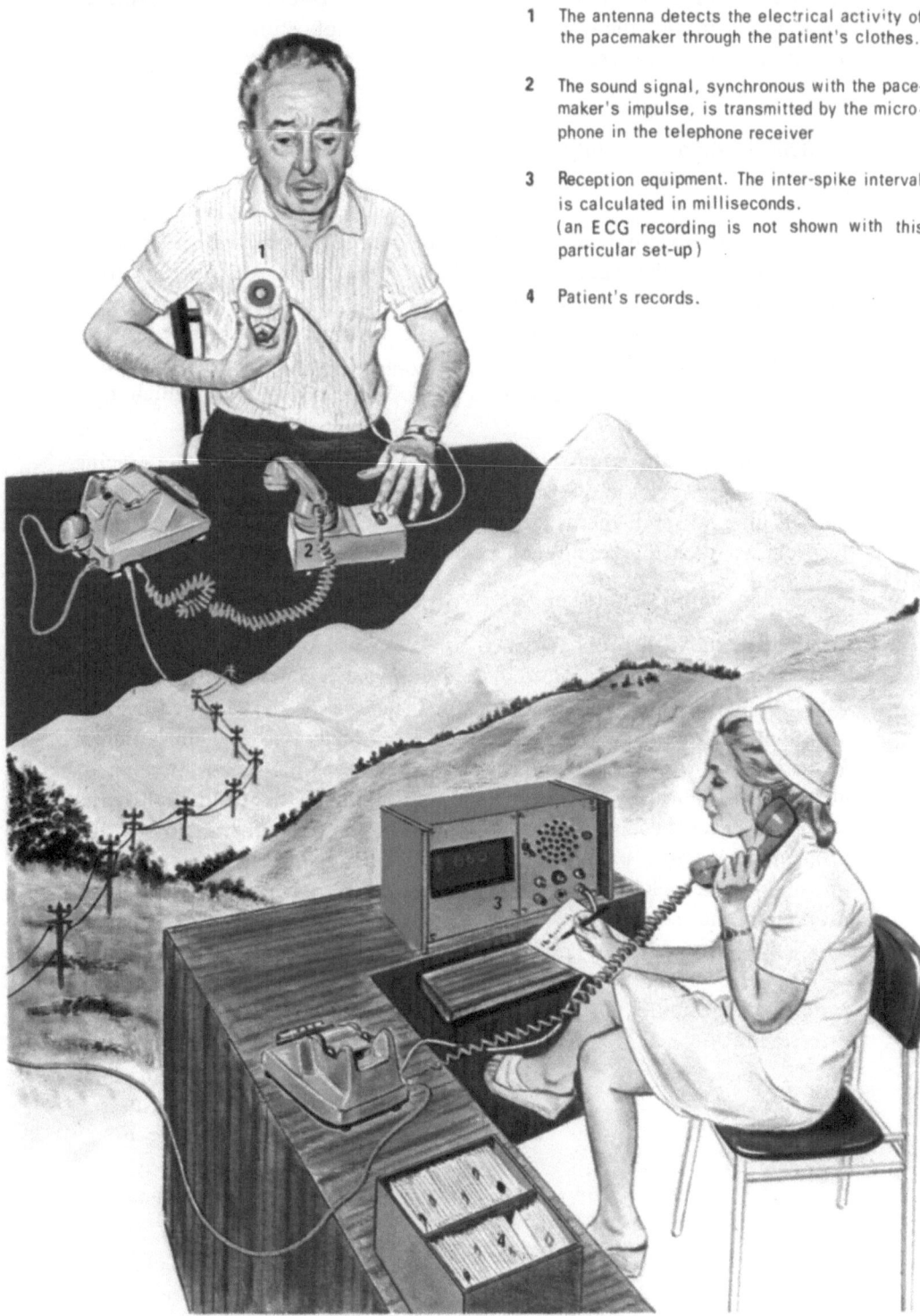

Tardieu

pacemaker has been in place, the result of the electrical measurements with and without the magnet, the duration of stimulations and its amplitude should be recorded.

g) **Follow-up by telephone**

This method is mainly used in countries where the patient lives a long way from the pacemaker centre (Plate XXIV, p 73). That is why it is mainly used in the Northern United States and in Canada. Differing systems are available. Some of them only transmit the impulse of stimulation which enables the period interval to be measured. Other devices are capable of transmitting not only the spike but also the patient's ECG. The underlying principle involves the amplification of the ECG as recorded between two arms, and transforming the electrical signals of the spike and QRS into a modulated frequency which may be sent by telephone.

A demodulation is carried out at the pacing centre and the tracing may be fed directly either to an electronic counter which shows the period interval and the frequency of stimulation, or on to a paper recorder so that the quality of pacing may be checked.

h) **Holter monitoring** (Plate XXII, p 65)

In patients with problems such as frequent unexplained blackouts a portable recorder may be used. Recording may sometimes last several days on a **cassette recorder** of the same type used to diagnose unexplained syncopes. When the tape is studied, two principle phenomena may be observed, either paroxysmal pacing faults, or periods of arrhythmias of varied nature which may explain the trouble. If the test is negative because the abnormality is too infrequent, and if the problem occurs in a patient who is pacemaker dependent, an exploratory operation to check on the pacing wires and their connections, their insulation and sealing and the screws of the pacemaker connections may be indicated. The threshold and endocavitary potentials should be measured using the pacing catheter. Only when all these results are negative, should the cause of the problem be attributed to another disease process.

REFERENCES

1. ANDERSON S.T., PITT A., WHITFORD J.A., DAVIS B.B. — Interference with function of unipolar pacemaker due to muscle potentials. *J. Thorac. Cardiovasc. Surg.*, **71**, 698, 1976.

2. BAROLD S.S. — Electrocardiographic diagnosis of myocardial infarction in patients with transvenous pacemakers. *J. Electrocardiol.*, **9**, 99, 1976.

3. BAROLD S.S. — Therapeutic uses of cardiac pacing tachyarrhythmias. In: «*His bundle*» electrocardiography and clinical electrophysiology - Narula O.S. Ed., *Davies F.A.*, Philadelphia, p. 407, 1975.

4. BAROLD S.S., GAIDULA J.J., CASTILLO R., MASOOD A., KELLER J.W. — Demand pacemaker arrhythmias. In: *Cardiac Arrhythmias*, Dreifus L.S., Likoff W. Ed. *Grune & Stratton*, New York 1973.

5. BAROLD S.S., PUPILLO G.A., GAIDULA J.J., LINHART J.W. — Chest wall stimulation of patients with implanted demand pacemakers. *Amer. J. Cardiol.*, **26**, 624, 1970.

6. BILITCH M., COSBY R.S., CAFFERKY E.A. — Ventricular fibrillation and competitive pacing. *N. Engl. J. Med.*, **276**, 598, 1967.

7. BILITCH M., LAU F.Y.K., COSBY R.S. — Demand pacemaker inhibition by radiofrequency signals. *Circulation*, **68**, 35, 1967.

8. BROOKS C., MAC C., HOFFMAN B.F., SUCKLING E.E. — Excitability of the heart. *Grune & Stratton*, New York, 1955.

9. BURCHELL H.B. — Analogy of electronic pacemaker and ventricular parasystole with observations of refractory period, supernormal phase and synchronization. *Circulation*, **27**, 878, 1963.

10. BUTTERWORTH J.S., J.S., POINDEXTER C.A. — Fusion beats and their relation to the syndrome of short P-R interval associated with a prolonged QRS complex. *Amer. Heart J.*, **28**, 149, 1944.

11. CAMMILLI L., BUTTINI C., POZZI R. — Radiofrequency cardiac pacing. *Ann. N. Y. Acad. Sci.*, **167**, 846, 1969.

12. CASTELLANOS A. JR, BERKOVITS B.V., CASTILLO C.A., BEFELER B. — Sextapolar catheter electrode for temporary sequential atrio-ventricular pacing. *Cardiovasc. Res.*, **8**, 712, 1974.

13. CASTELLANOS A. JR, LEMBERG L. — Electrophysiology of pacing and cardio-version. New York 1969, *Appleton Century Crofts*, p. 1.

14. CASTELLANOS A. JR, LEMBERG L., ARCEBAL A., BERKOVITS B., PIERETTI O.H. — Repetitive firing produced by pacemaker stimuli falling after the T-wave. *Amer. J. Cardiol.*, **25**, 247, 1970.

15. CENTER S., NATHAN D., CHANG Y.W. et al. — Two years of clinical experience with the synchronous pacer. *J. Thorac. Cardiovasc. Surg.*, **48**, 513, 1964.

16. CHARDACK W.M., GAGE A.A., FREDERICO A.J., SCHIMERT G., GREATBATCH W. — The long term treatment of complete heart block. *Prog. in Cardiovasc. Dis.*, **9**, 105, 1966.

17. CHATTERJEE K., HARRIS A., DAVIES G., LEATHAM A. — Electrocardiographic change subsequent to artificial ventricular depolarization. *Brit. Heart J.*, **31**, 770, 1969.

18. CHATTERJEE K., SUTTON R., DAVIES J.G. — Low intracardiac potentials in myocardial infarction as a cause of failure of inhibition of demand pacemaker. *Lancet*, **1**, 511, 1968.

19. CONDE C.A., LEPPO J., LIPSKI J. — Effectiveness of pacemaker treatment in the bradycardia tachycardia syndrome. *Amer. J. Cardiol.*, **32**, 209, 1973.

20. COUMEL P. — Different modes of pacemaking in the long term management of paroxysmal tachycardia. Symposium of cardiac arrhythmias. Sandoe E., Flensted Jensen E., Olensen K.H. Ed. *Astra*, Sweden, 783, 1970.

21. CRANEFIELD P.F. — The conduction of the cardiac impulse. The slow response and cardiac arrhythmias. *Futura publishing company*, Mount Kisco, N.Y., 1975.

22. DAMATO A.N., LAU S.H., BERKOWITZ W.D., ROSEN K.M., LISI K.R. — Recording of specialized conducting fibers (A-V Node, His bundle, and right bundle branch) in man using an electrode catheter tecnic. *Circulation*, **39**, 435, 1969.

23. DAVIDSON R.M., WALLACE A.G., SEALY W.C., GORDON M.S. — Electrically induced atrial tachycardia with block. -A therapeutic application of permanent radiofrequency atrial pacing. *Circulation*, **44**, 1014, 1971.

24. DAVIES J.G., SOWTON E. — Electrical threshold of the human heart. *Brit. Heart J.*, **28**, 231, 1966.

25. DE SANCTIS R.W. — Diagnostic and therapeutic uses of atrial pacing. *Circulation*, **43**, 748, 1971.

26. DREIFUS L.S., COHEN D. — Implanted pacemakers : medico legal implications. *Amer. J. Cardiol.*, **36**, 266, 1975.

27. DRILLER J.S., BAROLD S.S., PARSONNET V. — Normal and abnormal function of the pacemaker magnetic reed switch. *J. Electrocardiol.*, **9**, 283, 1976.

28. ESCHER D.J.W., FURMAN S., PARKER B., SOLOMON N., NAIDU S. — Computer analysis and telephone transmission of pacemaker artifact information. *Amer. J. Cardiol.*, **25**, 94, 1970.

29. EVANS T.R., CURRY P.V.L., FITCHETT D.H., KRIKLER D.M. — « Torsade de pointes » initiated by electrical ventricular stimulation. *J. Electrocardiol.*, **9**, 225, 1976.

30 FONTAINE G., KEVORKIAN M., WELTI J.J., RIBOT A., PETITOT C. — Comparison between endocardial versus myocardial and unipolar versus bipolar thresholds after long term pacing. In : *Cardiac Pacing* - Thalen Ed. *Van Gorcum*, Assen, 1973.

31. FRIESEN A., KLEIN G.J., KOSTUK W.J., AHUJA S.P. — Percutaneous insertion of permanent transvenous pacemaker electrode through the subclavian vein. *Can. J. Surg.*, **20**, 131, 1977.

32. FURMAN S. — Fundamentals of cardiac pacing. *Amer. Heart J.*, **73**, 261, 1967.

33. FURMAN S., ESCHER D.J.W. — Modern cardiac pacing (a clinical overview). *Charles Press.*, Philadelphia 1975.

34. FURMAN S., ESCHER D.J.W. — Principles and techniques of cardiac pacing. *Harper and Row.*, New York 1970.

35. FURMAN S., ESCHER D.J.W., PARKER B. — The pacemaker follow-up clinic. *Prog. Cardiovasc. Dis.*, **14**, 515, 1972.

36. FURMAN S., FISHER J.D. — Cardiac pacing and pacemakers. V - Technical aspects of implantation and equipment. *Amer. Heart J.*, **94**, 250, 1977.

37. FURMAN S., HURZELER P., DE CAPRIO V. Cardiac pacing and pacemakers. III - Sensing the cardiac electrogram. *Amer. Heart J.*, **93**, 794, 1977.

38. FURMAN S., PARKER B., ESCHER D.J.W. — Transtelephone pacemaker clinic. *J. Thorac. Cardiovascular Surg.*, **61**, 827, 1971.

39. GERBAUX A., LENEGRE J. — Observations sur les rythmes à double commande (sinusale et électrostimulation) constatés après implantation d'un stimulateur interne pour maladie d'Adams-Stokes. *Arch. Mal. Cœur*, **57**, 286, 1964.

40. GREEN G.D. — The assessment and performance of implanted cardiac pacemakers. London Butterworths, 1975.

41. GUSS S.B., KASTOR J.A., JOSEPHSON M.E., SCHARF D.L. — Human ventricular refractoriness : effects of cycle lenth pacing site and atropine. *Circulation*, **53**, 450, 1976.

42. HAAS J.M., STRAIT G.B. — Pacemaker induced cardio-vascular failure. Haemodynamic and angiographic observations. *Amer. J. Cardiol.*, **33**, 2, 295, 1974.

43. HAFT J.I. — Treatment of arrhythmias by intracardiac electrical stimulation. *Progr. Cardiovasc. Dis.*, **16**, 539, 1974.

44. HARTHORNE J.W., THALEN H.J. TH. — Boston colloquium on cardiac pacing. Martinus Nijhoff. The Hague the Netherlands 1977.

45. HARTZLER G.O. MALONEY J.D., CURTIS J.J., BARNHORST D.A. — Hemodynamic benefits of atrio-ventricular sequential pacing after cardiac surgery. *Amer. J. Cardiol.*, **40**, 232, 1977.

46. HOFFMAN B.F., CRANEFIELD P.F. — Electrophysiology of the heart. *Futura publishing company* - Mount Kisco N.Y. 1976.

47. IRNICH W. — Considerations in electrode design. In : *Cardiac Pacing* - Thalen H.J. TH. Ed., *Van Gorcum*, Assen the Netherlands, p. 272, 1973.

48. IWA T., WADA J. — Electrical and surgical treatment of tachycardias. In : *Cardiac Pacing* - Thalen H. J. TH. Ed. *Van Gorcum* Assen the Netherlands 1973. p. 376.

49. KARLOF I. — Haemodynamic effect of atrial triggered versus fixed rate pacing at rest and during exercise in complete heart block. *Acta Med. Scand.*, **197**, 195-206, 1975.

50. KARLOF I., BEVEGARD S., OVENFORS C.O. — Adaptation of left ventricle to sudden changes in heart rate in patient with artificial pacemakers. *Brit. Heart J.*, **38**, 537, 1976.

51. KASTOR J.A., DE SANCTIS R.W., LEINBACH R.C., HARTHORNE J.W., WOLFSON I.F. — Long term pervenous atrial pacing. *Circulation*, **40**, 535, 1969.

52. KASTOR J.A., LEINBACH R.C. — Pacemakers and their arrhythmias. *Progr. Cardiovasc. Dis.*, **13**, 240, 1970.

53. KENNELLY B.M., PILER L.W. – Management of infected transvenous permanent pacemakers. *Brit. Heart J.*, **36**, 1133, 1974.

54. KIDERA G.J. – Anti-hijacking devices don't affect pacemakers. *Jama*, **214**, 38, 1970.

55. KLEINERT M., BOCK M., WILHEMI F. — Clinical use of a new transvenous atrial head. *Amer. J. Cardiol.*, **40**, 237, 1977.

56. KRAMER D.H., MOSS A.J. — Permanent pervenous atrial pacing from the coronary vein. *Circulation*, **42**, 427, 1970.

57. KRIKLER D.M., CURRY P., BUFFET J. — Dual demand pacing for reciprocating atrioventricular tachycardia. *Brit. Heart J.*, **1**, 1114, 1976.

58. LANGENDORF R., PICK A. — Artificial pacing of the human heart. Its contribution to the understanding of the arrhythmias. *Amer J. Cardiol.*, **28**, 516, 1971.

59. LANGENDORF R., PICK A., WINTERNITZ M. — Mechanisms of intermittent ventricular bigeminy. I - Appearance of ectopic beats dependent upon the lenght of the ventricular cycle, the rule of bigeminy. *Circulation*, **11**, 422, 1955.

60. LEMBERG L., CASTELLANOS A. JR, BERKOVITS B.V. — Pacemaking on demand in A-V block. *Jama*, **191**, 12, 1965.

61. LINENTHAL A.J., ZOLL P.M. – Prevention of ventricular tachycardia and fibrillation by intravenous Isoproterenol and Epinephrine. *Circulation*, **27**, 5, 1963.

62. LISTER J.W., COHEN L.S., BERNSTEIN W.H., SAMET PH. — Treatment of supra-ventricular tachycardias by rapid atrial stimulation. *Circulation*, **38**, 1044, 1968.

63. LOWN B., KOSOWSKY B.D. — Artificial cardiac pacemakers. *N. Engl. J. Med.*, **283**, 907, 1970.

64. LUCERI R.M., FURMAN S., HURZELER P., ESCHER D.J.W. — Threshold behavior of electrodes in long-term ventricular pacing. *Amer. J. Cardiol.*, **40**, 184, 1977.

65. MANDEL W.J., LAKS M.M., OBAYASHI K. — Sinus-Node function : evaluation in patients with and without Sinus-Node disease. *Arch. Int. Med.*, **135**, 388, 1975.

66. MANDEL W.J., LAKS M.M., YAMAGUCHI I., FIELDS J., BERKOVITS B. — Recurrent reciprocating tachycardias in the WPW syndrome : control by the use of a scanning pacemaker. *Chest*, **69**, 769, 1976.

67. MEIBOM J. — « Vario-pacemaker », an implantable pacemaker especially designed for an easy check. In : *Cardiac Pacing* - Thalen Ed., *Van Gorcum*, Assen the Netherlands, 1973.

68. MELTZER L.E., KITCHELL J.R. — Cardiac pacing and cardioversion. *Charles Press*, Philadelphia 1971.

69. MOSS A.J. — Recent progress in cardiac pacing : therapeutic uses of permanent pervenous atrial pacemakers : a review. *J. Electrocardiol.*, **8**, 373, 1975.

70. MOSS A.J., RIVERS R.J., KRAMER D.H. — Permanent pervenous atrial pacing from the coronary vein.Circulation, **49**, 222, 1974.

71. NARULA O.S. — Atrio-ventricular conduction defects in patients with sinus bradycardia. Analysis by His bundle recordings. *Circulation*, **44**, 1096, 1971.

72. NARULA O.S. — His bundle electrocardiography and clinical electrophysiology. *F.A. Davis*, Philadelphia 1975.

73. NARULA O.S., RUNGE M., SAMEET P. — Second degree Wenckebach type AV block due to block within the atrium. *Brit. Heart. J.* **34**, 1127, 1972.

74. NARULA O.S., SAMET PH. — Right bundle branch block with normal left or right axis deviation. Analysis by His bundle recordings. *Ann. J. Med.*, **51**, 432, 1971.

75. NATHAN D.A., CENTER S., WU C.Y., KELLER W. — An implantable synchronous pacemaker for the long term correction of complete heart blok. *Circulation*, **27**, 682, 1963.

76. NOBLE D. — The initiation of the heart beat. *Clarendon Press*, Oxford 1975.

77. PARSONNET V. — A decade of permanent pacing of the heart. *Cardiovasc. Clin.*, **2**, 181, 1970.

78. PARSONNET V. — Permanent pacing of the heart : a comment on technique. *Amer. J. Cardiol.*, **36**, 268, 1975.

79. PARSONNET V., FURMAN S., SMYTH N.P.D. — Implantable cardiac pacemakers : status report and resource guideline. *Amer J. Cardiol.*, **34**, 487, 1974.

80. PARSONNET V., MANHARDT M. — Permanent pacing of the heart. *Amer. J. Cardiol.*, **39**, 250, 1977.

81. PARSONNET V., MYERS G.H., GILBERT L., ZUCKER I.R. — Prediction of impending pacemaker failure in a pacemaker clinic. *Amer. J. Cardiol.*, **25**, 311, 1970.

82. PRESTON T.A., BOWERS D.L. — Clinical applications of the threshold tracking pacemaker. *Amer. J. Cardiol.*, **36**, 322, 1975.

83. PRESTON T.A., FLETCHER R.D., LUCCHESI B.R., JUDGE R.D. — Changes in myocardial threshold - Physiological and pharmacologic factors in patients with implanted pacemakers. *Amer. Heart J.*, **74**, 235, 1967.

84. PUECH P. — Atrioventricular block : the value of intracardiac recordings. In : *Fundamentals of cardiac arrhythmias* - Krikler D. Ed.*Saunders*, London 1975.

85. ROBBOY S.J., HARTHORNE J.W., LEINBACH R.C., SANDERS C.A., AUSTEN W.G. — Autopsy findings with pervenous pacemakers. *Circulation*, **39**, 495, 1969.

86. ROSENBAUM M.B., ELIZARI M.V., LAZZARI J.O. — The hemiblocks. *Oldsmar. Tampa Tracings.* 1970.

87. RYAN G.F., EASLEY R.M., ZAROFE L.I. — Paradoxical use of a demand pacemaker in the treatment of supraventricular tachycardia due to the WPW syndrome : observation of termination of reciprocal rhythm. *Circulation*, **38**, 1037, 1968.

88. SAMET P. — Cardiac pacing. *Grune & Stratton*, New York 1973.

89. SCHALDACH M., FURMAN S. — Advances in pacemaker technology. *Springer-Verlag*, New York 1975.

90. SCHAMROTH L. — The disorders of cardiac rhythm. *Blackwell*, Oxford and Edimburgh 1971.

91. SCHEINMAN M.M., PETERS R.W., MODIN G., BRENNAN M., MIES C., O'YOUNG J. — Prognostic value of infranodal conduction time in patients with chronic bundle branch block. *Circulation*, **56**, 240, 1977.

92. SCHUILENBURG R.M., DURRER D. — Problems in the recognition of conduction disturbances in the His bundle. *Circulation*, **51**, 68, 1975.

93. SHORT D.S. — The syndrome of alternate tachycardia and bradycardia. *Brit. Heart J.*, **16**, 208, 1954.

94. SIDDONS H. — Deaths in long term paced patients. *Brit. Heart J.*, **36**, 1201, 1974.

95. SIDDONS H., SOWTON E. — Cardiac pacemakers. Springfield, Illinois, *Charles C. Thomas*, 1967.

96. SLAMA R., MOTTE G., COUMEL P. — Les blocs auriculo-ventriculaires. *Baillière*, Paris 1971.

97. SMIRK R.H., PALMER D.G. — Myocardial syndrome with particular reference in the occurence of sudden death and of premature systole interrupting antecedent T-waves. *Amer. J. Cardiol.*, **6**, 620, 1960.

98. SOWTON E. — Haemodynamic studies in patients with artificial pacemaker. *Brit. Heart.*, **26**, 737, 1964.

99. SOWTON E., BARR I. — Emergency management of patients with « Missed pacing ». *Amer. Heart J.*, **79**, 458, 1970.

100. SOWTON E., LEATHAM A., CARSON P. — The suppression of arrhythmias by artificial pacemaking. *Lancet*, **2**, 1098, 1964.

101. STARMER C.F., WHALEN R.E., MAC INTOSH H.D. — Hazards of electric shock in cardiology. *Amer. J. Cardiol.*, **14**, 537, 1964.

102. TAVEL M.E., FISCH C. — Repetitive ventricular arrhythmia resulting from artificial internal pacemaker. *Circulation*, **30**, 493, 1964.

103. THALEN H.J. TH. — Cardia pacing. *Van Gorgum*, Assen the Netherlands, 1973.

104. THALEN H.J. TH., VAN DEN BERG J.W., HOMAN VAN DER HEIDE J.N., NIEVEEN J. — The artificial cardiac pacemaker. *Van Gorcum*, Assen the Netherlands, 1970.

105. WATANABE Y. — Cardiac pacing. *Excerpta Medica*, Amsterdam 1977.

106. WELLENS H.J.J. — Contribution of cardiac pacing to our understanding of the WPW syndrome. *Brit. Heart J.*, **37**, 231, 1975.

107. WELLENS H.J.J., LIE K.I., DURRER D. — Further observations on ventricular tachycardias as studied by electrical stimulation of the heart. *Circulation*, **49**, 647, 1974.

108. WELTI J.J., FONTAINE G., BONNET M., KEVORKIAN M., PIOGER G. — Computer application for the control of an important group of pacemaker patients. In : *Cardiac Pacing* - Thalen Ed. *Van Gorcum*, Assen the Netherlands, 1973.

109. WIRTZFELD A., LAMPADIUS M., SCHMUCK L. — The influence of muscle potentials on synchronized pacemakers. In : « *Cardiac Pacing* » Thalen Ed., *Van Gorcum*, Assen the Netherlands, p. 169, 1973.

110. WYNANDS J.E. — Anesthesia for patients with heart block and artificial cardiac pacemakers. *Anesth. Analg.*, **55**, 626, 1976.

111. ZAKAUDIN V., MASON D.T., AWAN N.A., HILIARD G., MASSUMI R.A. — Lack of sensing by demand pacemakers due to intraventricular conduction defects. *Circulation*, **51**, 815, 1975.

112. ZIPES D.P., FESTOFF B., SCHAAL S.F., COX C., SEALY W.C., WALLACE A.G. — Treatment of ventricular arrhythmia by permanent atrial pacemaker and cardiac sympathectomy. *Ann. Intern. Med.*, **68**, 591, 1968.

TABLE OF PLATES